First

Spankings

First

Spankings

PETER BIRCH

Published by Accent Press Ltd – 2010

Print ISBN 9781907016271
Ebook ISPN 9781907726477

Printed and bound in the UK

Cover design by
Zipline Creative

Introduction

EVERYBODY REMEMBERS THEIR FIRST kiss. Everybody remembers how they lost their virginity. There's always something special about the first time, especially when it comes to sex. For some of us – and if you've picked up this book that probably includes you – another important milestone was the first time somebody smacked your bottom for you, or *vice versa*, your first spanking.

That is what this book is all about, first spankings – women's first spankings. These are not stories, but accounts of real spankings, most of them given by the women themselves. No doubt some cynical souls will dismiss that claim as improbable, even impossible, but that reflects only on their lack of imagination and experience. My fellow enthusiasts for the fine art of spanking girls' bottoms will recognise the situations and quite possibly some of those involved, although I have changed names and details when necessary in order to protect people's identity. It should go without saying that when I say spanking I mean erotic spanking between consenting adults, given and taken for the sake of sensual pleasure. Nor do I believe that it is in any way more appropriate for a woman to be spanked than a man, but as most people prefer one sex or the other to be on the receiving end I have stuck with my own preference.

For me, spanking is an essential part of sex. Without it sex lacks spice, and it is as important a part of foreplay as kissing. If that is incomprehensible to you, or seems in any way wrong, or you don't believe that women can, or should, enjoy spanking for the sake of sensual pleasure, then now

1

would be a good time to choose another book. It is not my intention to convert people, nor to explain myself in any way, but simply to entertain those who share my tastes. Nor do I intend to delve into the psychology of spanking, save in that these accounts contain a great deal of personal detail, with the same themes recurring again and again; the pleasure of submission, of shame, of exposure, or apprehension and even fear for those same emotions, often at the same time. That might seem contradictory, even impossible, but as any spanking enthusiast will tell you this is not the case, just the opposite in fact. Being spanked hurts and yet it is a thrilling sensation. Being spanked is highly embarrassing, humiliating even, and yet those very emotions can be gloriously arousing. Being spanked leaves you hot and sore, yet needing more of the same and needing sex. There is the need to be punished, the thrill of anticipation and apprehension, the fear of pain, the joy of pain, dozens of other emotions both raw and subtle. These are all facets in a complex whole, which you may have in greater or lesser degree, or not at all, so that despite these recurring themes no two people's experience and enjoyment are ever quite the same.

What I will do is provide a little advice. Perhaps most important, especially if you are the one doing the spanking, is that spanking is a mutual thing. You need to fulfil your partner's expectations as well as your own. Talk over your fantasies, discuss your limits and learn what's going on in each other's heads. You also need to respect each other's limits, while bearing in mind that those limits are never set in stone. Most importantly, if you're new together, or especially if you're introducing somebody to spanking for the first time, go easy. Many a promising situation has been ruined by the spanker wading in too hard, and I've known cases of both men and women with deep-set fantasies being put off the real thing by a clumsy introduction. The same goes for those on the receiving end, because it's surprisingly

2

easy to scare off an otherwise promising spanker by being too enthusiastic, especially when it comes to wanting punishment in front of other people.

There are plenty of books on technique, and this isn't intended as a guide, so I'm not going to go into that save for the most basic rule: avoid the bony bits, smack the plump bits. That's what bottoms are for, especially female bottoms, to provide a nice soft cushion, as well as attracting the boys, of course, and providing a source of arousal, which taken together make a woman's bottom not simply ideal for spanking, but the definitive target.

Spanking is also used as a punishment, and there's no denying the importance of that. Personally, I have always looked on spanking as both playful and erotic, and even now have little sympathy with the idea of punishment for its own sake. Not that I object to it, so long as the punishment is given with the full consent of whoever is receiving it, but for me there will always be a sexual element to spanking. In fact I admit to being sceptical of those who claim they give spankings purely as punishment or claim that they receive them purely as correction. What, with the woman bare bottom over the man's knee, every detail of her body on show and smacks being applied to a part of her anatomy as intimate as it is erotic? Even if you disapprove, surely you must see that as sexual?

Nevertheless, the punishment element is usually important and to many people crucial. The knowledge that you are giving or receiving a punishment can create powerful emotions, while the knowledge that one of you is entitled to punish the other is important in establishing the imbalance between spanker and spankee, which in turn drives much of the pleasure of submission. Hardly surprisingly, sexual display is the commonest recurring theme in these accounts of first spankings, but punishment comes a close second, and more often than not it is the need for punishment, genuine or contrived, that provides the

3

excuse for the spanking to be given.

As these are records of first times, the one giving the spanking was often older and more experienced, which is another important part of the spanking dynamic in any case, as the shyness and lack of confidence of the one being spanked adds to the thrill. The inexperience of many of those involved also means that in some cases things didn't go as smoothly as they might have done, so that some of the accounts have a clumsy feel to them or didn't work out the way one might have hoped. That's reality for you, and I can only hope that knowing these things really happened will make up for any lack of polish. You might also find the circumstances of some spankings mundane, but, again, that is reality. I have tried to include as much variety as possible, and rejected many otherwise perfectly good accounts simply because they mirrored others too closely, but you'll find no secret societies run by mysterious aristocrats, no lonely rural mansions where day to day corporal punishment is the norm, no perfect masters with harems of adoring slaves. Such scenarios are the stuff of fantasy.

What I do have for you are some wonderful experiences. The best spankings always have an edge, something that sets them apart, and I've focussed on those. Some come from my own experience, others were contributed by enthusiasts, but most accounts were taken as interviews with women who enjoy being spanked, conducted one to one and taken down longhand. All the content has been edited, but only to make the accounts easier to follow, rearranging events into the sequence in which they happened rather than in which they were told, adding those details essential to allow the reader to figure out what actually happened, and removing the ums and ers along with excursions into irrelevant subjects such as whether I'd like another coffee or the inevitable reminiscences of other spankings. As you can no doubt imagine, all this took months of work, but looking back, I wouldn't have missed a minute. In another sense it took

4

years of work, because not only have I recorded women's spankings dating back to the nineteen-thirties, but my own experiences across over thirty years.

Learning to Spank – my own account and several firsts

FOR AS LONG AS I can remember I always wanted to spank girls. It seems the natural thing to do with a pretty bottom, so much so that it never occurred to me for an instant that anybody might see things differently. For me, the desire to spank is as natural as the desire to kiss, and although I'm now wiser in the ways of the world I still find it impossible to see those who object to spanking as anything better than prudes and busybodies, just as I do those who object to kissing.

I suppose I was a late starter, at least by some standards, but with no sisters and having been at a single-sex public school from the age of seven I had very little contact with the female sex. That made my desire all the keener, but between my lack of company, my unorthodox sexual tastes and a body like a bag of coat hangers it took a while before I found myself a regular girlfriend.

Oh, and one important point. I was never beaten at school, and for me at least there is no correlation whatsoever between having to endure the threat of being hit with a stick by some mouldering old sadist and wanting to smack girls' bottoms as erotic play. The beautiful and alluring junior matron on the other hand … but never mind that, back to my first real girlfriend.

Two Ferrets in a Sack – Debbie Swann

The first girl I ever spanked was also the first girl to spank me, for the simple reason that she was only prepared to accept what I would take in return. That struck me as fair then and it still does now. Tastes vary, but I've always felt it unreasonable, even dishonourable, to refuse to accept what I'm so eager to dish out. I enjoy it too, but that's not the point.

Debbie and I were both spankings virgins. I don't think it had even occurred to her that spanking could be sexual, although she was very aware, and proud, of her bottom. She wiggled so nicely when she walked that she used to compare her rear view to two ferrets fighting in a sack. She was very slim, with small, oval cheeks and rather soft flesh, hence the wiggle. I wanted to spank her the moment I saw her, but then that's hardly unusual. I was also drawn to her beautiful auburn hair, which fell almost to the back of her knees, and her cheeky, vivacious character. She was also very open and made no secret of her feelings for me, which at the time was exactly what I needed.

We used to joke about spanking, but when I suggested she deserved it she would always try to turn the tables on me rather than teasing until she got it, which is what any real enthusiast would have done. And yet she was always keen to experiment sexually, with different positions and techniques, even with attention to her bottom hole. In the end I simply told her that it was going to happen, that her knickers were coming down as well as her jeans, which were already around her knees at the time, and that I was going to smack her bottom with a ruler. This was in my bedroom, with me sitting on the bed and her standing in front of me, her blouse open and her bra lifted over her breasts, her jeans pulled down as I kissed and licked at her body. She said she'd let me do it, as long as I would accept the same from her. At the time it had never really occurred to me that I, or any man,

7

might be on the receiving end of an erotic spanking, but I agreed, both on principle and because at that moment I'd have cheerfully agreed to go off in search of the Holy Grail if it meant she'd allow me to smack her wriggly little bottom.

Given my lack of experience, and that for her it wasn't even a special fantasy, I think it went rather well, although giving a spanking is definitely something that takes practice and this was my first time. Yet it was something I thought about every day and I'd devoured every scrap of literature on the subject that I could find, even if it was all muddled together in my head. That's probably why I didn't put her across my knee, but instead told her to put her hands on top of her head. She obeyed, a little reluctant and perhaps having difficulty trying to accept erotic embarrassment as sex play for the first time in her life, but truly beautiful with her breasts peeping out from between the edges of her blouse and her expression ever so slightly sulky as I turned down her knickers to bare her back and front.

I turned her around, leaving her neat little bottom just a foot in front of my face as I picked up the ruler from my desk. For years the idea of having a girl present me with her bare bottom to spank had been my favourite fantasy, so the excitement of the moment was almost overwhelming and has left a clear impression in my mind. I remember smacking the ruler across her cheeks, hard, how her soft, pale flesh bulged above and below the wood, and the faint red impression it left. It wasn't very hard at all, but it made her squeak and after the second smack she asked me to stop. I put the ruler down and kissed her bottom, pressing my lips once to each cheek where the pink flush showed, then began to caress her and use my hand to pat her gently.

Debbie didn't seem to mind that, and at last I was spanking a properly compliant girl. Just to have her like that would have been enough for me, to feel my fingers on the softness of her flesh and watch the way her cheeks quivered

8

to the slaps. She had even pushed her bottom out a little, treating me to a hint of the tight, pink dimple of her anus and the rear of her sex lips. It was a view I'd imagined a thousand times, and admired in a hundred pictures, a spanked girl seen from the rear, and I could have carried on all day. Unfortunately she was growing increasingly embarrassed and fidgety, demanding that I take my turn, although to be fair she didn't try to move but stayed just as she was, bare bottom and with her hands on her head, until I finally relented.

She used the ruler on me, in the same position more or less, and curiously my reactions were very similar to her own, perhaps typical of somebody who is willing to play but is having trouble coming to terms with their feelings. The ruler stung too, and I can sympathise with her objecting to having it applied to her virgin cheeks.

After that first episode spanking became a regular thing between us, although she was always the one on the receiving end. My willingness to accept it if she asked was enough to satisfy her pride. She got quite into it, or at least used to it, and certainly appreciated my attention to her bottom. Unfortunately we lived too far apart for our relationship to work at all well, and with hindsight I realise that we're weren't really all that compatible. Nevertheless, she was my first, as I was hers, losing our virginities to each other as well as experimenting with spanking. There will always be a special place for her in my heart, and for that glorious moment when I turned down her knickers and took my old school ruler to her bare bottom.

The second girl I spanked, the first of three called Jane, was more experienced than me and used to get dealt with by her regular boyfriend, but she deserves a mention because it was playing with her that removed the lasts traces of doubt from my mind that girls like it too. Debbie was always a little shy, a little hesitant, and I could never quite rid myself of the suspicion that she only gave in to please me, despite her protestations to the contrary. Jane was very different, especially the first time, giggling at my request and presenting her bare bottom in a delightful kneeling position on my bed, then purring happily as I smacked her full, pale cheeks up to a glowing pink. She was plump, and that's not intended to be disparaging as I find voluptuous women every bit as attractive as their slender sisters. That's especially true when it comes to spanking, because a big, meaty bottom has a beauty all its own and is always a delight to play with. Jane's certainly was, full and firm with skin like cream, while her favourite kneeling position made her hips flair and exaggerated the size of both her bottom and her breasts, which were also large and very full. Unfortunately our liaisons were brief and on her part guilty, as while I thought she'd broken up with her boyfriend they were still seeing each other. When he proposed to her she broke off our relationship, and that was that. It was to be quite some time before I got to dish out another spanking.

Spanking Angst – Beth Wood

Beth was only the third girl I ever spanked, but it was her first time and the memory is still fresh in my mind. I met her before either Debbie or Jane, and I'd always found her fascinating, because of her pretty, up-turned nose and the splash of freckles across her cheeks, because of the long, brown hair that fell to her waist in luxurious curls, but most of all because of her bottom. She was gloriously well built, with a slim waist and hourglass hips that accentuated full, heavy cheeks more often than not packed into tight blue jeans or a pair of burgundy-coloured cords she had which were so tight and so revealing that she seemed not so much to be wearing them as upholstered in them. Just to watch her walk used to make my mouth dry, while to follow her up the steep stairs that led to her flat was enough to leave me badly in need of a cold shower. She was also nice; fun, sympathetic and easy going, but sadly for me – a gawky bespectacled student – her taste in men ran to something more rugged.

I was of course more than just a gawky bespectacled student. I was a gawky bespectacled student with somewhat peculiar sexual tastes, but she didn't know that. Or maybe she did, because several other people knew by then and these things do tend to get around. If she did, then she kept it to herself, and it didn't seem to affect her attitude towards me. What she did know was that I was in love with her, and while she was sweet and understanding she'd made it very plain that we could only ever be friends.

So friends we stayed. At first that was excruciatingly painful emotionally, especially as when she ran into difficulties with the various Neanderthals she liked to go out with it was always me she came to for the male perspective. Looking back, we were actually quite physical. We'd hold hands, kiss, cuddle a little, enough to give one or two of the Neanderthals the wrong idea, but that was it and I wanted more. Above all I wanted to get to grips with her lovely bottom; to kiss her cheeks, to bury my face in the deep cleft between, and of course, to spank her.

In the end it happened, and it only happened because I physically could not resist her. We were at my house, quite late, with nobody else about, just watching the television. I can picture her exactly. She was face down on the floor, her chin propped in her hands and her legs kicked up, one shoe dangling negligently from her toes. Her top was cream-coloured and printed with big, red flowers, poppies I think, very 70s, and she had on her burgundy cords, leaving her bottom a perfect ball of cheeky girl flesh between the gentle curve of her back and her thighs. I wanted to touch her so badly it hurt, and in the three years I'd known her by then, I'd never quite given up hope, so I asked her, jokingly, if I could use her as a pillow. To my surprise she said yes, and so I laid my head on her bottom.

I expected her to tell me to get off, in that same gentle, understanding tone she always used if she felt our cuddles were going a little too far. She didn't. I stayed as I was, hardly daring to move, but drinking in her perfume and luxuriating in the meaty softness of her bottom flesh. I could have cried, and it took all my will power not to stick my hands down the front of my trousers then and there. She carried on chatting and watching the television, as if nothing out of the ordinary was happening.

Even heaven loses it's initial thrill eventually, but it must have been 15 or 20 minutes before I dared to move a little, with the pretence of making myself more comfortable as I put one arm across her thighs and shifted my head further onto her bottom. Again I expected her to object and again she didn't react at all. I had to touch, even if it meant I got a lecture, just to feel the curve of that glorious bottom for one fleeting instant.

I did it, making a joke about how comfortable she was as I plumped up her cheeks as if she'd been a real pillow. She felt so good, soft yet firm, exquisitely feminine and so, so spankable. Now I was sure I'd pushed it too far, but she just laughed, and when I kept my hand on the curve of her cheek she made no objection. I began to stroke, lost in bliss as I explored the curves of her bottom, expecting to be told to stop it an any moment, but that moment never came. Slowly I grew bolder, lifting my head so that I could touch her properly and see what I was doing. I began to squeeze, and to trace my fingers down the narrow valley where her cords followed the curve of her cheeks down into her crease.

She'd stopped talking. There was no more pretence about what I was doing. She obviously didn't mind me fondling her bottom, perhaps because she liked it and knew she could tell me to stop whenever she wanted, perhaps because she knew how desperately I wanted her and felt sorry for me. Perhaps she didn't even see what I was doing as a sexual

12

thing. I didn't ask and I didn't care. All that mattered was the feel of her cheeks and that if I was allowed to stroke then possibly, just possibly, she wouldn't mind a gentle pat.

Again I screwed up my courage and did what I needed to do so badly. My touches turned to pats, very gentle ones delivered to the tuck of her cheeks. Still she didn't respond, so I began to pat a little harder and to my amazement she lifted her bottom, offering me her cheeks. So I spanked her. It wasn't hard, and I never even tried to get her trousers down, let alone her knickers, but it went on for a long time, with her bottom pushed right up, full and round in those skin-tight cords, my pats turning gradually to smacks and always alternated with strokes and squeezes to her flesh. She let me kiss her bottom too, just on the seat of her cords, and rub my face against her, all of it without either of us ever saying a single word.

How far we might have gone I don't know, but I suspect that if I'd tried to unbutton her trousers or pulled up her blouse it would have broken the spell, or maybe not. I'll never know, because after I'd been playing with her for maybe half an hour my parents came back and that was that. I thought that after what had happened there was something between us at last, but when I spoke to her the next morning I was given that same sweet but firm refusal and we never mentioned the incident again. Even now I don't pretend to understand what was going through her head, but I certainly know what was going through mine and the incident has been a happy memory ever since. It was an important milestone in my spanking career, because for the first time I had enjoyed giving a spanking for its own sake rather than as part of foreplay. I won't say that she opened my eyes to the possibility of having spanking partners without any other sexual contact, but looking back she was my first spanking playmate.

Beauty in Abundance – Rhiannon O'Brian

My second, spanking playmate, and my first regular one, was Rhiannon O'Brian, an Irish girl I'd met shortly before going up to university and whom I remained friends with for several years. Rhiannon was a big girl in every sense, as voluptuous as she was voluble, always talking and always laughing, which would make her chest shake in a manner calculated to bring tears to the eyes of a statue. Her breasts were huge, and for her age, gigantic, each so big it took both hands to hold properly, also round and firm. Not surprisingly she was used to male attention, and she expected it, but when we first met I had other things on my mind, mainly Beth.

Had I shown interest in Rhiannon I expect I would have joined her long list of unsuccessful admirers. She was a terrible flirt, with the ability to keep men hanging on for months, even years, in the hope of her showing them favour for the simple reason that sometimes she actually would. I don't suppose it was calculated. She liked male attention and she liked sex, so if she happened to be with somebody at the right time and in the right place she would have him, and it was very much a case of her having him. Some got lucky, more didn't, but she always made it very plain that she didn't belong to anybody.

The one thing guaranteed to earn her contempt was to crawl after her, especially for those she'd already had sex with. I was the exact opposite, usually reserved, and when I did open up it would be to bemoan my lack of success with Beth. Rhiannon put up with this for over a year before one memorable and drunken night at her parents' house. The details are a little hazy, but I remember that I'd come straight there from college, cycling some eight miles from central London, and that the first glass of ice-cold cider barely seemed to touch the sides of my throat. I remember her asking me why I didn't find her attractive, and although

14

I can't remember what I said in reply she seemed to take it as a provocation. I remember her lifting her top and bra to invite me to admire her chest, but that may have been later, and I remember her delight as I lost myself in pleasure over her breasts, although I suspect that the red-blooded male who wouldn't has yet to be born. I remember her crawling along the floor, naked, with her full bottom lifted and open, an irresistible target.

What she expected was sex. What she got was a spanking. Why she didn't get both I'm not at all sure, but this was the early 80s and we didn't have any condoms, so maybe I was simply following government advice. In any case I took her around the waist and spanked her bottom. She was big and firm, very meaty, and compared with both Jane and especially Debbie seemed to be capable of soaking up an awful lot of punishment. I did it really hard, and she absolutely revelled in it, despite it being her first time, which I didn't know. Her reaction only encouraged me, to the point where my hand was stinging with pain and her entire bottom was a rich red. I'd have given her more, if I'd had an implement to hand, again my memory is hazy as to the exact sequence of events, but I do remember her hand on my erection as we lay in bed together later that night, and a peculiar conversation about my respect for her, or lack of it, as she masturbated me.

After that night spankings became a regular occurrence for her. She was always very shy about it, insisting that we keep it between ourselves, and on calling the shots. Not that I minded, because if we were alone together, especially if we hadn't seen each other for some time, the chances were that she would end up with a hot red bottom, and quite possibly with my cock in her hand. That was as far as we ever went, and it was a fairly strange relationship by most standards, but for me the first of a great many like it, and my experiences with her did teach me one very valuable lesson: that men and women can be friends and have sex at the same time, or at least, kinky sex.

Who Needs Privacy? – Miranda & my second Jane

Two other girls deserve a mention from the very beginning of my spanking career, Miranda and my second Jane. Both took their first spanking from me and both also gave me a new first; Miranda because she was the first girl I spanked in front of somebody else, and Jane because she was the first girl I spanked outdoors. Both spankings occurred as part of brief and unsuccessful liaisons, and within a few weeks of each other.

Miranda was an old school friend of my cousin, Kirsty, who we'll come back to later. We met on a night out not much different to dozens of others, with a group of friends meeting up in a pub before returning to my cousin's house. Miranda seemed keen on my company, and before long we were kissing on Kirsty's bed. I've always had an exhibitionist streak, although not so much for showing off myself as for showing off any girl I happen to be with, while I knew that Kirsty and the others wouldn't mind in the slightest. Soon I had Miranda's top up and her tiny, firm breasts naked in my hands. She didn't mind, and if anything seemed rather proud of herself, so that when Kirsty offered us the chance to spend the night on her floor we accepted.

What followed would have been a typical one-night stand, the sort of thing everybody has done many times, except that Kirsty was enjoying the view as Miranda and I stripped each other down, and the spanking. Miranda was small and neatly built, her bottom round and high. I was kneeling on the floor as I took her jeans and panties down, and while I hadn't specifically intended to spank her, having her bare in my hands made it the natural thing to do, so I buried my face between her thighs and gave her several firm swats while I licked. She'd never been licked before, let alone spanked, as I learnt the following day when she

16

explained that I wasn't "man enough" for her, as if cunnilingus followed by letting her go on top so that I could hold her warm bottom as we had sex made me effeminate! I hate to think what she'd have thought if I'd asked her to spank me.

My encounter with my second Jane started in much the same way. I forget how we met, but it was one evening on the town among many, and again she was keen on my company, attention I was more than happy to accept. There the resemblance ends, as she was far more innocent than Miranda and definitely not up for sex on our first night. She was eager enough, but still a virgin and determined to remain that way, so that for me it was like being a teenager again. I'd have called it off, except that there was something about her – call it chemistry – that drove me nuts. She wasn't exceptionally attractive, although she did have a fine chest, but just to hold her in my arms was enough to leave me achingly hard. Up until then I'd thought of the idea of a woman giving a man "relief" as a clumsy euphemism for sex, but all of a sudden I understood it, and I needed it.

Three times I ended up going home in such a state that only by the exercise of every last ounce of my willpower did I hold back from risking arrest for gross indecency on a public omnibus, but on the fourth occasion it was just too much. We'd walked up to her uncle's allotment for some privacy, and I was sitting on an old wooden packing case in the angle between his shed and a hedge. Jane was on my lap. We were quite invisible, so she'd let me pull her top and bra up so that I could play with her lovely breasts as we kissed. She was in jeans, and I knew that to try and undo them would be going too far, but that didn't stop me squeezing and stroking her bottom, which she didn't seem to mind. I felt ready to burst and put my hand to my zip, only for her to tell me not to be dirty, an extraordinary statement for a girl with her boobs bare and her nipples not only stiff but wet from sucking. So I told her we'd try something else and I

17

bent her down across my knee, as much out of sheer frustration as my desire to spank her. To my surprise she didn't seem to mind, giggling as I smacked her bottom, so I tucked her up tight, with one arm around her waist and went to town on her, smacking her cheeks hard enough to make my hand sting and set her legs kicking.

She took it well, and it may be that she was used to it, although she later claimed it was her first time. Her bottom looked glorious too, tight in her faded blue jeans, and to cap it all the way she was tucked up across one leg meant that my cock was rubbing on the softness of her thighs through our clothes. Every smack to her bottom gave me just a little friction, and while she must have realised she didn't protest, just wriggling a little and kicking her feet as I spanked her, giggling between playful squeals. I kept her there for ages, enjoying her bum and hoping the rubbing on my cock would take me over the edge, but I couldn't quite make it. In the end I simply couldn't hold back any more. Tumbling her off my lap, I unzipped and finished myself off by hand in front of her as she sat there, her eyes wide and her mouth open in shock, her lovely breasts still bare and, at the end, also distinctly messy.

We lasted another three weeks after that, and she was also the first girl I spanked at college, kneeling on the floor of my room with her nightie up under her arms so that I could play with her breasts while I smacked her across the seat of her knickers. Afterwards she let me come between her breasts but that was as far as it went and she never could quite handle the strength of my desire for her. She is now a senior police officer.

College Spankings – a few more from the vaults

COLLEGE AND SPANKING GO well together. Girls in mini-skirts or skin-tight trousers, little round bottoms on top of long, coltish legs, a touch of innocence and a touch of naughtiness, it's the stuff of fantasy. Reality, sadly, seldom quite comes up to the mark, but by a combination of obsessive determination and boundless optimism I managed to have a pretty good time during my four years as a student.

From a spanker's point of view my first year at university was backward looking and outward looking. With the exception of the second Jane all my encounters had taken place at home, and not a single one of my fellow students had felt the sting of my hand across her bottom. In my second year that was to change completely.

In Search of Times Past – Felicity South

I had opted to live out of college, in a shared house convenient for the science area but also used to accommodate the overspill from the main hall of residence. Felicity had the room below me. She was exceptionally petite, with a delicate oval face framed by copper-coloured hair cut into a neat bob, big grey-green eyes and delicate lips that seemed to be forever slightly parted. I fell in love with her at first sight, both for her shy, vulnerable beauty and her exquisitely English charm, and the robust attitude I'd begun to build up towards my female friends vanished in an instant.

19

Looking back, I was far too circumspect with Felicity, too cautious of her bad opinion and not nearly bold enough, but I did at least get to spank her, eventually. Like my second Jane, Felicity was a virgin, but unlike Jane she unmanned me completely. We were together for six months, but while we were intimate enough in our way I could never break through her reserve, nor show her the physical passion that might have made the difference. Even now I can only conjure up one good erotic image of her, as she was when I called in late one night, in nothing but a light cotton nightie that hinted at the dark triangle of hair between her thighs and the sweetly turned curves of her breasts and belly, her hips and bottom. She had no knickers on.

That image stayed with me long after we'd given up on what was obviously a hopeless relationship, each to move on to a new partner. We remained friends, but seldom saw each other, and more seldom still once I had gone down from university. Occasionally a snippet of news would reach me, which was how I learnt that she had married the new man in her life and, just two years later, got divorced, which was how matters stood when I met her at a college fundraising event. Neither of us knew anybody else there at all well, so it was only natural that we sat together for a dinner that saw one excellent wine follow the next across six courses. The idea was presumably to lubricate the guests into being generous with their donations, but it certainly had the effect of lubricating Felicity into being generous with her body. Long before we got up from table her eyes were bright with pleasure in a way I'd never seen while we were together, and we were kissing the moment we could find a dark nook. I'd have had her then and there, if she'd let me, and quite probably caused an impressive scandal, but she at least had the sense to make me wait until we were back in her guest room.

Once the door was closed everything that should have happened in our six months together happened in the space of about six minutes. She was in a pretty blue gown, which came off over her head within seconds, leaving her naked but for her heels and tights, also blue, and her panties. We went down on the sofa, kissing, touching without inhibition, and before long she was straddled across my lap with her back to me and her bottom pushed out so that she could rub herself on my erect cock, presumably a trick her husband had taught her, because I certainly hadn't.

By that point spanking was such a familiar part of sex for me that I never thought to question whether she'd appreciate it or not. With her lovely little bottom rubbing on my erection she was not going to escape unsmacked. I tipped her forward and pulled down her tights and panties as one, baring her for the first time. She was fleshier than she had been, more womanly, but all the better for that, and her cheeks bounced beautifully as I began to smack them, turn and turn about, to make her gasp, still wriggling her bottom onto my cock before lifting herself onto me and sinking down with a long, contented sigh.

Her tights and panties were making it difficult to fuck and she'd quickly peeled them off, leaving her nude and me still in full black tie, immaculate save for the exposure of my cock and balls. I carried on spanking her, enjoying the view of my cock inside her and the tight pink dimple of her anus between her red cheeks, even wondering if I dared try and put it up her bottom, but with that thought I realised I was going to come. Despite the drink and the ecstasy of my approaching orgasm I managed to lift her off before it was too late, tipping her forward onto the floor and finishing myself off over her now well spanked bottom instead of inside her.

We sat up for hours, first with her laid still naked across my knees as I rubbed hand cream into her smacked cheeks and brought her off with my fingers, then side by side on the sofa. It was light by the time I left, after she had confessed that while her husband had gone some way to teaching her

21

to appreciate her body, and in particular her bottom, she had never been spanked before, but wasn't in the least surprised that I'd wanted to do it to her. Evidently she knew me better than I'd realised.

Hair – my third Jane

I'm not entirely sure about this one, as it was a brief encounter and I never got around to asking her if she'd ever been spanked before. Judging by her reaction I'm fairly sure she hadn't, but you never know. I was still in my second year at college and she was the younger sister of one of my housemates, Alison, whom she'd come up to visit. We went out in a large group, about twelve of us, to visit the Penultimate Picture Palace on the Cowley Road, I think, although for all I can remember of the evening it might as well have been the Hanging Gardens of Babylon. Jane showed an interest in me from the start, at which I was surprised, flattered and not a little guilty, because while my relationship with Felicity was obviously hopeless we were still together at least in name.

Jane was quite tall, had exceptionally long legs and a small, round bottom, but her most striking feature was her hair, which was Nordic blonde and worn in a single plait that fell to her ankles. Apparently it had never been cut, which I could easily believe, and she was proud of it and pleased by my appreciation. She was also very frank and open, which at the time made a pleasant change, and even suggested that we might go up to her sister's room, but on the understanding that I shouldn't expect sex. I wasn't entirely sure what she meant, but as we'd already been kissing and cuddling I knew that at the least she had no objection to me touching her bottom, so accepted after only a moment of guilty hesitation.

She was a joy, easy-going and confident in her body, out of her clothes almost before we'd got the door safely locked and just as keen to get me out of mine. I was soon pulling her hair as we played together, something she was particularly keen on, and as I was answering her needs it seemed only fair that she should answer mine. So I asked if she'd mind a gentle spanking, only to have her react in shock and surprise. I spent the next couple of minutes explaining that what I actually wanted to do was smack her bottom, which included some wonderful lines on her part, delivered with a truly delightful combination of astonishment and innocence, something like –

"On my bottom? What, like I've been a naughty girl?"
"If you like, or just for fun."
"For fun? You like to smack girls' bottoms for fun?"
"For you as well. It'll feel nice."
"Having my bottom smacked!?"
"Yes. Come on, let me show you. I'll pull your hair while I do it."

That got to her, and she finally complied, doubtfully, although she did ask me what position I'd like her to be in. We were on the bed, so I had her kneel, twisting the long braid of her hair into my fist as I set to work on her bottom, stroking and kneading her flesh before I began to spank her, very gently at first. She was shaking, and kept glancing back at me, her face full of doubt, but I continued to pull at her hair and smack at her cheeks. Her skin was exceptionally pale, and soon began to grow pink, while with my hand locked tight in her hair she had little choice but to arch her back, allowing her cheeks to come open and show off her anus and the rear of her pussy. She was already wet, and getting wetter as I warmed her bottom, with beads of moisture growing at the mouth of her sex, while there was no mistaking the implication of the sighs and moans escaping her lips, nor the change in her breathing. I still held back, making the smacks harder only very gradually, but all the time wishing I had three hands so that I could look after myself as well as her.

She could see the effect she was having on me though, and finally twisted around to take me in her hand, tugging so enthusiastically it hurt. I continued to spank her, properly now, really enjoying her bottom and the thought that I was being masturbated by a girl as she knelt in the nude while her bottom was smacked, something that just moments before she'd thought of as only suitable for a punishment. I came in her hand, then went down on her to return the favour, only to have her sister knock on the door before we'd finished. Sadly that was the only time I ever saw her, but the incident led on to other things, several months later.

A Spanking Earned – Violet Chertsey

Violet was in the year below me and a close friend of another of my housemates. When I first met her she seemed painfully shy, but we slowly got to know one another better, until by the end of my second year we'd developed a strange but intimate relationship. We used to cuddle, and she'd cling on to me like a drowning kitten while I treated myself to a leisurely exploration of her neat little bottom. I never did give her what I'd consider a proper spanking, but she knew what I was like and loved to lie over my knees to have her bottom patted and stroked. That was it, because she made it plain where the limits lay and I respected them. I didn't even see her nude until years later.

At the time I simply accepted what was admittedly a rather unconventional relationship at face value. What she really wanted was just to be held, but she liked her bottom stroked, I liked to stroke her bottom, each of us giving the other what they needed. She knew that I'd have loved to take down her panties and spank her properly, but I accepted that it wasn't going to happen. It did occur to me to wonder whether she used to play with herself afterwards in the quiet and privacy of her own bed, but it seemed rude to ask.

She's now married and a successful career woman in her own right, but we still see each other occasionally and get on very well, so that when I told her I was writing this book she agreed to provide me with some background detail. Violet –

"I found it soothing with you, like a massage. I knew you wouldn't try to take advantage, and it was nice."

"Most people would say …"

"I know. That it was inappropriate touching, or something like that. I'm not most people. You were my friend, and you liked to pet my bottom, so why not?"

"To pet your bottom. That's a nice way of putting it, and you're right. I wouldn't have taken advantage, even if you'd let me spank you properly."

"You did spank me. You used to spend ages spanking me!"

"I mean harder, and on your bare bottom."

"Bare skin would have been too intimate. Maybe on my knickers."

I hate it when girls says things like that. On one occasion I'd played with her while she was in just knickers underneath her nightie, and the thought that she wouldn't have minded having it turned up gave me a sharp pang of regret. The next thing she said surprised me.

"Besides, it hurts bare."

"So you have been spanked? I mean, by somebody else. Don't tell me Michael spanks you?"

"No! He'd be horrified."

"Who then?"

"Donald."

"Before we met, your first boyfriend?"

25

"Yes."

"Do you mind telling me about it?"

"I suppose not. It was when we were going out. He always used to say he was going to do it, but I wouldn't let him. Then after we came back one night, from a fair in Stockport, he said it was time I was spanked. I asked him why and he said it was because I needed it, so I told him not to be stupid. Why did I need to be spanked?"

"And why did you?"

"I didn't! He just wanted to spank me, that's all."

"That's understandable. But you wouldn't let him?"

"No. It wasn't that I minded, so much, but I didn't want to be spanked for nothing. I didn't want my spanking to be unimportant. He was always complaining that I took my time getting ready, so I told him he could do it if I was ever more than an hour late to go out."

"So you could tease him, or did you intend to be deliberately late?"

"No, neither! I was very careful not to be late after that."

"But you'd admitted you had a spanking coming to you under the right circumstances?"

"No. I accepted that he could do it if I deserved it."

"But you admit the possibility of you deserving a spanking?"

"Yes, if you want to put it like that."

"It's important. Who admits they deserve a spanking unless it's what they really want?"

"Me ... okay, I admit I quite liked the idea of him punishing me. This is embarrassing, Peter."

"Take your time."

"Okay. In the end I was late because I missed a bus. We were going to a friend's party and I had to get to his house first so another friend could take us by car. When I got there he was the only one left. I was genuinely sorry, but I'd forgotten all about my promise, until he told me to come upstairs. I thought he was after a kiss and a cuddle, so I told him it could wait, but he said I was to be spanked."

"So you let him?"

"No, not right away. I put up a real fuss, but he wouldn't budge. In the end he picked me up over his shoulder and took me into the living room. I was still trying to make excuses as he put me over his knee, and I was struggling. It took him ages to get my party dress up and pull my knickers down, but as soon as I was bare I stopped fighting. I don't know why."

"And he spanked you?"

"Really hard. It hurt so much and I felt so ashamed of myself I thought I'd choke, but he was determined to get through to me."

"To punish you? So he did actually feel you needed to be spanked?"

"No. It was what turned him on, and he was sure it would do the same for me. It did. When he'd finished I let him … you know. Afterwards he told me what he meant by saying I needed spanking, not to punish me, but to turn me on."

"And he was right."

Her answer was a nod and her face was the colour of a beetroot, so I decided I'd pushed her far enough. She had rather opened my eyes anyway, because all the time I'd known her I'd assumed that she was a virgin, at least until she got engaged to Michael and probably until her wedding night, and I would never have guessed that Donald had spanked her.

Striking Gold – Penny Smith

Violet was the eighth girl I'd spanked, as Felicity came later, and in every single case I had been the driving force behind what happened, with the girls more or less compliant but never the instigators. With Penny it was a different matter entirely, because while she'd never been spanked before her fantasies made mine look tame. Penny –

"If you read my first collection of short stories, 'Bad Penny', you'll find a story called 'Pretty in Pink', in which I'm given my first ever spanking by my Aunt Elaine at my cousin's wedding, in my pink bridesmaid's dress but panties down and over her knee, of course. That's a favourite variation on my original spanking fantasy, but while the details change the ingredients are always the same; being brought down to size, going from being fully dressed to completely exposed, and being spanked harder than I can cope with. It's really all about humiliation for me, you see, so in a way the reality was better than the fantasy. After all, you could argue that my aunt has a right to spank me, and so I should accept it, but not from some toff in a dinner jacket!"

Penny and I were in different years and studying different subjects, I lived out of college and she lived in, and we moved in very different sets, so we would probably never have met had it not been for a particularly fine piece of irony. Unknown to me, my third Jane had told her sister about her spanking. Alison had been horrified, to put it mildly, not only branding me a pervert and an abuser but somehow managing to work in the huge chip she carried on her shoulder about social class, although never in a million years would it have occurred to me that I wanted to spank

Jane as some sort of bizarre gambit in a class war, or even to punish her for being insufficiently servile, although the idea does have its appeal. I do like a nice maid, preferably OTK with her frilly knickers pulled down.

To Alison I was the enemy. Not only did I come from a public school background, but I indulged in just the sort of bizarre sexual behaviour she would have expected, and with her little sister. Since learning what I had done with Jane she had lost few opportunities to blacken my name, although she was always pleasant enough to my face and I was blissfully unaware of what was going on. I'd had similar problems as a teenager, picking up a reputation for pervy behaviour with the local girls which put most of them off but always intrigued the rare few with unconventional tastes. The same now happened again, because while no doubt the great majority of Alison's friends shared her delighted disgust at the knowledge that one of the public school men in college liked to spank girls, one didn't, little Penny Smith. Her reaction was rather different –

"I was completely fascinated. I knew men like you existed, but I'd assumed they'd be older, maybe a tutor or something. That's what I used to fantasise about anyway, but it would never have happened. Nobody could admit to that sort of thing, and I certainly couldn't! Most of my friends were second-generation feminists, and there I was wanting my bare bottom spanked, so you can imagine how careful I was to keep my feelings to myself. The way Alison reacted, anybody would have thought you were a serial rapist at the very least. It would never have occurred to her that I didn't feel the same way, and I certainly wasn't going to admit to the truth. So I pretended to be shocked and disgusted while I milked all the juicy details out of her, about how you'd made Jane kneel on the bed in the nude and wanked off while you spanked her."

"She had me in her hand, and she was pretty keen."

"That detail got lost somewhere in the telling. The way I heard it you were really pervy with her, telling her she had a pretty bumhole and how her pussy showed from behind."

"I suppose I might have said that. I remember how she looked."

"Exactly how I wanted a man to see me, only over his knee, always over his knee. I must have come over that thought a hundred times, and ever time I saw you around college it made my bum tingle in anticipation. I thought you were really brave too, for going through with your fantasies, because I would never have dared unless I was one hundred per cent sure of getting the right reaction."

"You had some bad experiences, didn't you?"

"More frustrating. I always used to hope somebody would spank me, but they never did. I couldn't have asked for it straight out, never, and my subtle hints just didn't seem to sink in."

"Give me a couple of examples."

"Alright. There was Rick, who I don't think you ever met. When I pretended that the boy I'd been out with before had threatened to spank me he said he'd hunt him down and beat him up, not the reaction I wanted at all! I didn't try that one again, and when I suggested to Stephen that maybe it wasn't such a bad thing if girls were given corporal punishment occasionally he gave me a long lecture about his respect for women. I think he thought I was trying to catch him out."

"So for all your fantasies you'd never been spanked?"

"No, not unless you count self-spanking?"

"No. That's just you, darling."

In fact it's not, as I know plenty of girls who started with self-spanking, and quite a few who still do it if there's nobody around to oblige, but while it can be difficult to define what does or does not count as a spanking I do think somebody else has to be involved, even if it's only to turn on the spanking machine, but we'll come back to that later. Penny had managed to reach her first year of university without being spanked, despite it being a desire so strong that it dominated her sexuality. The knowledge that there was a man in college who not only liked to spank girls but had actually done so, and in her friend's room, made me irresistible.

I had no idea any of this was going on. My relationship with Felicity was over in all but name, while I had Rhiannon to spank at home and Violet at college, not an ideal situation but not a bad one to be in by any means, especially after years of struggling to find the right girl for my tastes. I'd seen Penny around college but I didn't even know her name, although I do remember admiring her long, dark hair and the way her bottom filled out the rather tatty jeans she used to wear. The only other thing I remember about her from that period is that she tended to walk around as if she was in a world of her own. This was a marked improvement on her friends, most of who seemed to cultivate an identical, disapproving scowl with which to face the world.

There were certainly a few scowls when she joined the college wine society, of which I was president at the time. I had been trying to get more women to join, leading Violet to joke that "Peter wants more women", so I was only mildly surprised, and took care to welcome her as I would have any other new member who wasn't already close friends with the established set. She began to come to tastings, but was always very quiet and shy, although fairly knowledgeable, as her elder brother proved to be in the trade. Then came the annual dinner, an extravagant affair of twelve courses, each accompanied by at least two suitable wines. I had sat Violet

31

to my right as my choice for female company, but when we finally retired to drink brandy and smoke cigars it was Penny who came to talk to me. The rest of the evening is somewhat hazy for me, but she had drunk far less and remembers what happened in detail. Penny –

"I'd never been so bold in my life, but I knew you liked to spank girls so I didn't see why you shouldn't want to spank me, especially after a dinner like that. I'd even dressed on the assumption you'd be seeing my underwear, in tarty red knickers that tied up in a bow at either hip."

"Those I do remember, under your subfusc, such a contrast."

"I thought I looked a complete frump, but my subfusc was the only thing I had for a dinner. I couldn't afford an evening gown. I even had to think twice about the knickers. They cost six quid."

"Worth every penny. So you came to talk to me after the dinner?"

"Yes. I thought you had something with Violet. You did, sort of, but I thought you'd be going to bed together, the way you'd been talking all evening, so when she left early I saw my chance. I felt really guilty, but the thought that you might spank me was too good to resist, so I was telling myself the spanking would be a punishment for going behind her back. That turned me on so much, and once we'd got talking it all just seemed to happen. You said you'd walk me back to my room, and then we were kissing in the doorway. You put your hands on my bum and gave me a little pat, and I just melted. You knew exactly what to do, and you were so firm about it, shutting the door and leading me over to my big chair, kissing me and touching me up, and then you bent me over the chair. That was when I knew it was really going to happen. I was going to get spanked. You knew exactly how to handle me."

"I was drunk. Just following my instincts."

"Which were to bend me over my own chair and pull up my skirt for spanking! That was bliss. I remember the way you did it, with one hand around my waist to keep me from getting up as you tugged up my skirt. I was in black stockings and one of those little frilly suspender belts they used to sell in the 80s, wasn't I? I was sure you'd like that, but I was panicking about my knickers. I was sure you'd think I was a tart for wearing them, but all you said was – 'Very cute.' And then you'd started to rub my bottom through them."

"That's another clear memory, pulling up your skirt to find your panties barely covered your bottom. You were spilling out at the sides, and the back was lacy anyway, so I could see the crease of your bottom."

"I know. I'd been looking at myself in the mirror before I came out, thinking what a little tart I looked and how I'd like to be spanked for that. I'd never wanted it so badly in my life, and it's something I used to fantasise over every single day. I swear I nearly fainted when you finally stopped feeling me up through my knickers and pulled open the bows at the sides. They just fell down, and all of a sudden my bottom was bare. Being bared, that's another of my favourite things. It felt so indecent like that, with my skirt rolled up and my big, fat, white bottom sticking out …"

"You were rather neat and trim, actually, fleshy maybe, but not fat."

"I know, but when my bottom's bare and I'm going to be spanked I love to think I'm fat, and you're thinking what a little porker I am as you feel my cheeks up. It's more humiliating that way. You really got to me too, the way you put your hand on my bottom and gave my flesh a wobble, then pulled my cheeks apart so you could inspect my bumhole. You took ages, and I was wondering if you minded me being so hairy, and if you could see how wet I was, and how hard you were going to spank me. Then you tightened your grip on my waist and you started, using your fingertips to make it sting, then your cupped hand so the smacks were really noisy. I was sure my neighbours would hear and know I was getting a spanking, which was just so humiliating, but I had just enough common sense to ask you to try and be less noisy. You told me to shut up."

"Sorry."

"No. It was perfect. You went back to using your fingertips, but I felt so completely humiliated, thinking of Mary and Alison coming in and catching me with my tarty little panties undone and my fat white bottom stuck out with my pussy and bumhole on show while you spanked me. I just had to come."

"I fell in love with you when I saw that you were playing with yourself. That was perfect."

"For me too. You kept on spanking while I did it and you were calling me a bad girl and telling me I deserved what I was getting and how you ought to do it in public. That was too much. I was thinking of you spanking me in front of all my friends, their horror and my total humiliation as I got it bare bum in front of them. I came, and then you made me suck you off."

"Just that?"

"No. It's a bit intimate … oh, what the hell. I didn't even realise you'd got your cock out until you stuck it in my mouth. I'd never sucked a man before, but you

34

didn't know that, of course, and I was desperately trying to pretend I was experienced, only when you went back behind me I had to say it, because I was scared you'd hurt me. I was babbling out that I was a virgin, but you'd already got your cock to my pussy hole and I could feeling my hymen stretching, and then it had burst. God that stung so much, but you'd pushed really hard and your cock had gone right up me, only it really hurt and I was begging you to take it out. I didn't think you would, because you were right up and obviously needed to finish off, but you were really sweet, dirty though. 'Okay, I'll do it in your mouth then', that's what you said, and you did, making me suck my own cream and my virgin blood off your cock while you wanked in my mouth, you filthy pig!"

"It was too good to resist."

So was she, and with the start of our relationship my life changed completely. Following my relationship with Felicity I had promised myself that I would never again accept a relationship that wasn't openly and frankly sexual. That I got with Penny, who took to sex like a Russian to vodka, but always with at least a little spanking first. I was in heaven, and made a thorough pig of myself, spanking her at every opportunity. Penny –

"I remember walking up the river to the Victoria Arms. I think you must have had me bend over every stile and every fence we crossed, not to mention making me touch my toes in the middle of a field, and walk with my knickers turned down. That's worse than having to go bare, as if anybody does see they know I'm showing off on purpose, otherwise I might just be in a G-string. Then there was the Chinese food fight in the punt, when you ending up putting a load of sweet and sour pork balls down my knickers and spanking me like that. I think I put that in one of the Isabelle books, or maybe Penny Pieces. Most of the things we did ended up in print, including the episode with the chocolates and my bottom hole."

"Yes, only you made your partner a muscular black rower."

"A girl can dream, and anyway, you're the one who got your cock dirty."

I had, giving her a first taste of anal sex with the aid of half a box of molten chocolate creams, which remains among the messiest things we've ever done. I had never realised a girl could be so filthy, and we encouraged each other, swapping fantasies and then acting them out. As she says, most of what we did has ended up in her books, often with very few details changed. For instance, her affair with her cousin Kate is loosely based on her first lesbian experiences, only the girl involved wasn't her own cousin, but mine. Penny had always enjoyed the thought of sex with another woman, and particularly being spanked –

"I used to fantasise about the blonde girl in a certain 70s pop group. She had a lovely bottom, and I used to imagine being put across her knee for a bit of discipline and then being made to kiss her bum to show how low I was next to her. Naturally that got ruder, until it used to be my tongue up her bottom and … well, you know."

"Yes, I do. You really are an absolute disgrace. But what about Kirsty?"

"Oh yes. You were always trying to get her to spank me, weren't you? She wasn't really into it, was she, but she liked me and in the end she did me just to keep you happy, and because she knew how much it would turn me on. It was in her bedroom, wasn't it, with you holding my knickers down at the back while she smacked my cheeks. The best thing was knowing it was another girl doing it, and because she's taller and slimmer than me. That's another favourite of mine, being spanked by a group of fashion models for having the nerve to compare myself with them. They'd strip me first, stark naked, and pass me around between them for spankings, with me on my knees as I crawled from one to the next, then make me lick them out, one by one, kiss their bumholes and finally put me in the middle of a circle and piss all over me."

"Great, but you were telling me about Kirsty?"

"Yes. That was my first spanking from another woman, but not the last."

It wasn't, not by a very long way indeed. To find that my new girlfriend was not only a true spanking enthusiast but bisexual was a dream come true, while she was more than happy for our relationship to include other people, at home or away, so long as we stuck to two basic rules: no emotional involvement, and nobody whose intention is to come between us. I could not have asked for more, and so, reader, I married her.

Spanking Good Times – old friends, and family

GETTING TOGETHER WITH PENNY marked the end of my formative years as a spanker. The hard work was done, the chase won. I now had the loveliest girl I could possibly have imagined to spank more or less when and where I pleased, subject to the usual constraints such as being considerate to her feelings of the moment or not doing her in front of her family. Doing her in front of my own family was a different matter, as we have seen, but it went rather further than that.

Strip Poker – Kirsty Graham

It is with some trepidation that I admit to spanking my own cousin. Not that I can see any reason why I shouldn't, as she was old enough at the time and definitely consenting, but some people are funny about that sort of thing and it's easy to imagine the raised eyebrows and the disapproving thoughts. Then again I'm used to that and she is lovely, a natural blonde with a willowy, almost elfin figure, also very much a free spirit and a born exhibitionist. She used to strip for me, purely for fun, and out in the countryside it was hard to get her to keep her clothes on at all, which led to an amusing incident with a tractor driver on one occasion, but that's another story. Her bottom is small and tight, perhaps not ideal spanking material but nevertheless irresistible when offered with the words "Go on then, spank me if you have to." So I did. It's probably just as well I don't have any sisters.

That was long after her first time, but it was probably only the fourth or fifth. She wasn't into it, but she'd known I was ever since the incident with Miranda, while of course she'd spanked Penny and I'd spanked Penny in front of her on more than one occasion, knickers down too, so she could guess that I'd happily give her the same treatment. She liked the exhibitionist element, particularly the idea of being held in place while her bottom was exposed, but not the pain. So despite the intimacy between us I had always held off, contenting myself with what she chose to give, and that was plenty. Then came the time the three of us were playing bondage games in her bedroom. Penny had already been dealt with and was running around naked from the waist down with her red cheeks peeping out from under her top, so it was Kirsty's turn. We tied her hands behind her back and took down her jeans and knickers, with her lying face down on the bed. Her bottom looked deliciously inviting, a neat, pale little peach with a wisp of honey blonde hair showing between her thighs. I wanted to smack it, my natural reaction to a girl's bare bottom, or a girl's clothed bottom for that matter, and Kirsty knew perfectly well I wanted to smack it, hence her offer. We shared her, a cheek each, and got her quite pink before she decided she'd had enough.

Her first spanking had come several years before, during a game of strip poker. She had been playing with her boyfriend of the time, his brother and girlfriend and another couple who'd been to the same school. I suppose it was typical of that sort of thing, plenty of drink and six young people all keen to see their friends' partners stripped down, although apparently it was a regular occurrence for the other two couples but the first time Kirsty and her boyfriend had been involved. Kirsty –

"They were seriously out to get me, most of all Merrick, maybe because I was his big brother's girlfriend, or just because I was older, because the

39

girls were nearly as bad. I think they were cheating anyway, because I was the first one to have to take my top off and I was in the nude before any of them were really showing anything. I was getting that tingly feeling, and it was really turning me on being nude in front of them, so when Lindy said that if I lost again it would have to be forfeits I said I was up for it. I lost and they made me stand up with my hands on my head and turn around really slowly so they could all have a good look, then when I lost again somebody suggested I ought to be spanked, Lindy again I think. The others thought it was really funny, so I said they could as long as it wasn't too hard. So Evan made me bend over one of the armchairs and the others got round behind so they could all watch. He made me stick my bum right out so they could see everything and he smacked me with Lindy's hairbrush. It really hurt, but I let him give me six so it wouldn't look like I was trying to back out or anything."

"Maybe if he'd been a bit more gentle you'd have enjoyed it more?"

"Maybe. It's not so bad when it's with a hand, but I just hate pain."

"Fair enough. And afterwards? You mentioned before that your spanking was the highlight of the game."

"That was nice. I felt sort of warm and comfy, and really horny. Evan took me to bed and we had the best sex."

"So it wasn't all bad?"

"No. I do like it, being stripped bare and having to stick it out to be smacked, and the warm feeling, but you have to be gentle with me."

Which I have tried to be on the handful of occasions I've spanked her, and which illustrates an important lesson from the introduction, that if you want to initiate somebody into spanking you should always start gently, especially if they don't already have the fantasy in their head.

A Sharp Lesson – Jasmine Drake

Jasmine is an old friend of Penny's; very slim, with blonde curls and a bouncy little bottom. I first spanked her side by side with Penny in the back of the old estate car I owned at the time, with both girls bent over the rear seats so that they could see each other's faces and the various dirty old men lurking in the shadows of what was one of London's most notorious dogging car parks at the time. I took down their jeans and knickers and spanked them both well, enjoying not only the delightful view they were giving me but their embarrassment as they were spanked in front of each other. Not that it was our first time out dogging, and I have many a happy memory of sitting between the two of them with their tops pulled up as they enjoyed themselves with my cock and balls. Nor was it the first time Jasmine had been spanked, but she was relatively innocent and more used to dishing it out than getting it, hence her remark, delivered in a wonderfully sulky tone of voice as I pulled down the little green panties she was wearing "I thought it was the boys who got spanked?".

That was her experience, up until then, with one important exception, but it's worth recording the aftermath of that session in the car park before moving on. She'd bought a two litre bottle of cider to keep us warm for the evening, but Penny hardly drinks and I was driving. Jasmine had already drunk quite a lot in order to pluck up the courage to show off in public, and even then it took us a while to persuade her to join Penny over the back seat for a spanking. Once I'd got her bottom warm it was a very different matter. She wanted more, and she wanted as many people as possible to see. After what I'd done to them I was

41

already fit to burst, so I had them sit either side of me to finish me off in their hands and mouths, as we'd done before, but still with their jeans down and a hot bottom in either hand. Jasmine was playing a dirty trick, taking swigs of still cold cider and going down on my cock with her mouth full, which was bliss and had inevitable consequences. By the time she'd got the taste out of her mouth with yet more cider she was very drunk and wanted to be spanked over the bonnet of the car. There were several other cars there and quite a few single men, so I could see things getting badly out of hand. We told her to play with herself in the back instead, which she did, finishing the last of the cider as she lay spread out with her top pulled high and her fingers busy between her legs. By the time she came there were men all round the car, and I think at least one or two women from other cars, but we had the interior light on and could see them only as moving shadows, a strange experience. Unfortunately one man got too insistent, banging on the window and demanding that Jasmine suck him off. He wouldn't take no for an answer, so we drove away. By the time we got back to her place Jasmine was asleep, and so drunk I had to help her indoors.

We saw her again two days later. She was delighted by what we'd done and up for more, but we soon realised that she couldn't remember what had happened after her spanking, except that there'd been other people around and that I'd been talking to somebody in a serious voice. In a moment of supreme mischief Penny began to pretend that we'd been caught by a constable and that I'd only managed to get us out of trouble by promising him the girls would go round to his house for sex. Penny said that she'd already been, that the policeman had spanked her and made me watch while she sucked his cock. It was a typical Penny fantasy, especially the details such as having to do it kneeling and with her jeans and knickers still down so that her smacked bottom showed, but to my astonishment

Jasmine not only fell for it but allowed Penny to persuade her that if she didn't do the same the police would be around her house later that same evening. I couldn't help but join in, and we got Jasmine as far as being about to ring the bell of a completely random house before we admitted that we'd made it all up. Fortunately she has a good sense of humour.

Jasmine was always receptive to new ideas, and nobody could call her narrow-minded. Her first spanking had come about a year before the car park incident, at the hands of a local call-girl. Linda worked out of a flat in Jasmine's road and they had been at the same school, although three or four years apart. They'd meet occasionally, and while Jasmine's ambition in life was to find a worthwhile man and start a family she was tempted by Linda's lifestyle, while the idea of sex for money didn't bother her in the slightest as long as she didn't have to go all the way.

Some of Linda's clients liked to be beaten, and one in particular had a fantasy about being watched, and sneered at, while he was punished. He was prepared to pay well, and when Linda asked Jasmine if she'd help out they quickly reached an agreement. Jasmine was rather good at sneering, partly because she had a naturally mocking laugh, and partly because she genuinely found the sight of the man on his knees as Linda applied a cane to his buttocks funny. He appreciated the attention and after two or three session asked if Jasmine would cane him too. She'd happily have done it, but Linda insisted on making a new booking, for the following week.

When Jasmine arrived the next week she was very surprised indeed to be told that if she was to cane the man she would have to learn how it felt. Being Jasmine she quickly allowed herself to be talked into it and ended up being taken up to Linda's bedroom to learn how it felt to be beaten. Standing by Linda's bed, she was made to turn up the short, tight denim skirt she'd put on for the session and had her knickers pulled down. Her bottom was smacked, first in the standing position and then bent over the bed, before she had six cane strokes laid across her bare cheeks. She says it didn't hurt all that much, and I suspect Linda was quite gentle. I also suspect that Linda had no interest whatsoever in teaching Jasmine how it felt, but simply wanted to spank and cane her friend without admitting to lesbian feelings.

A Hint of Fetish – Dusk & Silke

Two other old friends deserve a mention, although sadly we've lost touch with both and so I was unable to gather the details of their first spankings, at least with any certainty.

I taught evening classes on wine appreciation in Camden at the time, and while I was used to a pretty varied collection of students, one stood out in a way I considered both eccentric and erotic. She was always immaculate, her dark hair brushed and coiled and pinned into one exotic style or another, her make-up as elaborate and striking as it was unusual, and she wore black leather. Her three-quarter length, military-cut coat, her knee length, high-heeled boots, her tiny dresses that left the full length of her thighs on show, all were black leather. If she happened to be walking up the stair in front of me – something that seemed to happen surprisingly often – I'd be treated to a glimpse of snugly fitting black panties, and on at least one occasion those were also leather.

She called herself Dusk, almost certainly not her real name, and my initial guess was that she was a high class call-girl who specialised in men with exotic tastes and was attending my classes in order to improve her knowledge of fine wine and therefore her skills as a hostess. That intrigued me, especially as her dress suggested that spanking might well be included in her repertoire, if only dishing it out. Not that I had either the need or the money for her presumably expensive services, but I suspected that she might be a

44

kindred spirit.

Unfortunately I was wrong on both counts. By the end of the year I knew her quite well, enough to discover that she wasn't a call-girl at all, but simply a near terminal fashion victim who worked in one of the trendy shops nearby, while the nearest she'd come to getting a spanking was the playful application of a friend's riding crop to the seat of her skin-tight black leather trousers. That may well have been her first, and she wasn't in the least reticent about it, just not into it, or anything else kinky apart from dressing up, so far as I know. No doubt she made a great partner for the right man, or woman, but I'd been hoping for a new playmate and that clearly wasn't going to happen.

Her friend was another matter. She was German, called Silke, shared a flat with Dusk, and came from the Mosel wine country. We hit if off immediately, with plenty in common, although I was a little cautious at first, because given Dusk's exaggerated femininity and Silke's short cropped, ash-blonde hair and taste for tatty clothes and steel-toed work boots I assumed that they were lesbians. Again I was wrong, she quickly become firm friends with Penny and myself, and, unlike her friend, she proved to be actively kinky. I suppose I should have guessed from Dusk's admission about the riding crop, which was done as a game one night when Silke was going out to a club and had to wait what she considered an unreasonably long time to use the bathroom. Dusk came out, fully dressed in her leather finery, and was told to present her bottom for being a naughty girl. She obliged, sticking it out for a half-dozen or so gentle strokes with Silke's riding crop, which given the way her bottom filled her leathers must have been a sight worth seeing, however casual.

Knowing that Silke had taken an active pleasure in applying a riding crop to her friend's bottom made her easier than ever to talk to. We began to swap stories, sitting in a dingy, old-fashioned pub somewhere at the back of Camden

45

and trying to outdo each other for outrageous behaviour. One of Silke's stories included what may well have been her first spanking, and is well worth setting down in any case. The house where she'd been brought up was on the edge of one of the Mosel's most famous wine villages, with the bottom of the steep, slate vineyards coming right up to the wall at the end of her parents' garden. All her life she had been a dedicated scrumper, slipping over the wall on quiet autumn evenings to feast on the ripe Riesling grapes. More than once she'd been spotted and chased, but she was too edgy and too agile to be caught, while in a large village full of little blonde girls it wasn't hard to avoid identification. Nevertheless, there was suspicion, as she discovered when she returned home after her first year of study in England. Spurred on as much by nostalgia and several cool beers as by any desire to steal grapes, she once more slipped over the wall, to walk up between the long rows of vines, sampling the occasional grape. Unfortunately she had abandoned her childish caution and on reaching the top of the row found herself face to face with the grower himself, who had ducked down among the vines either to inspect his crop or because he'd seen her coming. Either way he recognised her and immediately launched into a lecture, the gist of which was that she ought to know better at her age. As she had grape juice running down her chin she could hardly deny her crime, but being Silke, she simply laughed at him, stuck out her bottom and asked what he was going to do, spank her? To her amazement he did exactly that, planting one hard smack full across the seat of her jeans and a second to her thigh as she dodged away. At the time it was a shock, and she gave him the full benefit of her opinion as she fled, but she also admits that she found the memory of that smack and the sting of her bottom afterwards shamefully arousing. So, not much of a spanking, but it does conjure up a beautiful picture.

The reason Silke was carrying a riding crop the night she

whipped Dusk was that the club she was going to was Der Putsch, London's foremost fetish club at the time, where a small group of dedicated enthusiasts would meet once a month for kinky and clandestine games. Silke not only admitted this to us, but suggested that we should go. It had never really occurred to me that there might be a community of people like myself and Penny. I knew about spanking magazines and videos, but I had always assumed that was commercial and that as a man my involvement was unlikely to go beyond being charged extortionate prices for second-rate goods. The existence of a club like Der Putsch opened a whole new world of possibilities, but what with one thing and another we never got there. We went to Skin Two instead, and Submission, and Torture Garden, and within a year of meeting Silke we were regulars on the London Fetish scene.

A Pervert's Paradise – spanking accounts from fetish friends

OUR INTRODUCTION TO THE fetish scene marked another sharp change in my spanking career. We'd spent the previous six years playing with a small, close group of friends, and when it came to the spanking we were very much the driving force. All that time had been Penny the only woman I knew who craved spanking rather than simply enjoying it if it happened to be on the menu or being prepared to accept it as part and parcel of playful sex. That now ceased to be true.

London's fetish scene is paradise for a spanker, or a pervert, as we quickly came to call ourselves in ironic reference to the way we were treated by the media. Not everybody who's involved in fetish may be into spanking, by a long way, but in a fetish environment you are free to ask without the risk of causing offence, and while the answer will often be no, it will also often be yes. It wasn't so much that we'd tasted honey and sought for more, as that we'd discovered a large vat of the stuff and not merely eaten it but immersed ourselves up to our necks. Of the two hundred or so people we've spanked or been spanked by between us, more than half have also been involved with the fetish scene in one way or another, so readers will have to excuse me if things now get a little less domestic and a little more kinky.

Over Uncle Colin's Knee – Charlotte York

Penny and I had been on the fetish scene for a short while when we met Charlotte, who was the first fetish girl I spanked and went on to become one of our most intimate playmates. I remember the event well, a private party at a cottage deep in the countryside and only a short distance from my old school. Even after a dozen years it felt both strange and exhilarating to be attending a fetish party at a place I'd often walked past when sneaking in with drink or simply trying to escape the tedious routines of boarding school for a few hours. We'd also driven straight from Devon, picking up a new riding crop and five metres of chain on the way, so we were in a good mood and ready to play. It proved to be quite a night, and although we only knew a few of the other people there everybody was very friendly and our hosts were careful to make all the proper introductions. The only ones I remember are Charlotte herself – small, trim and pretty with an appealing timid look – and her enormous Scots boyfriend, Rory – six foot plus with a beard like a haystack. My first impression was that this was how a master and his slave ought to look.

Later that evening we were delighted to find that Charlotte's timid appearance hid an inner fire and an almost insatiable appetite for corporal punishment. She loved to be spanked, paddled, whipped and generally taken to task with any implement to hand, while she also loved to go nude. She was being spanked over her boyfriend's lap while the rest of us were still chatting, but it wasn't long before the party had got going in earnest. The cottage was pretty small, but they'd still managed to find space for a windowless "dungeon" with mirrored walls, an astonishing range of bondage and punishment equipment, and a curious device like a medieval cannon carriage only padded with leather and hung about with chain, ropes and a complicated system of pulleys – the bondage horse.

The horse was soon being put to good use by our friends Natalie and Gemma, both of whom you'll meet later. Both were usually dominant, but at private parties it was a very different story, with Natalie allowing her strong submissive streak to show through. Gemma soon had Natalie strapped to the horse, her nipples clamped and chained, her bottom stripped for the attention of a vicious little dog whip. The rest of us watched entranced, growing slowly more aroused, until one by one the couples began to play, at first together and then more or less at random. My memory of the rest of the evening is hazy to say the least, but includes licking wine off one girl's bare breasts, having crushed ice applied to my own burning buttocks after a whipping from another girl, Charlotte pulling down Penny's little blue panties to spank her, and she getting hers in turn, across our linked knees with her legs kicking and her bottom pushing up in her mingled pain and ecstasy. I think we may have used a hairbrush.

That was the first of many encounters. The four of us got on well, with similar tastes and boundaries for what was and was not acceptable. Over the years I've probably spanked Charlotte more often than anybody else except Penny, but I still relish the thought. Not only is she pretty and a lot of fun, but sweet and tart at the same time, while she has a trim figure and pale skin with the texture of cream, so lovely that when she's bare over my knee I can never decide whether I'd rather spank her or just stroke her bottom. I usually manage both.

I've known about her first spanking for a long time, as she told me the story one day as we walked back to her boyfriend's flat after a long and alcoholic lunch. Like so many girls, she'd been angling for it long before she actually got it, and, also like many girls, it was important to her not to have to ask for it right out. She used to tease, to show off her bottom in skin-tight jeans or mini-skirts with little white panties underneath, to cheek her boyfriends and hint that she deserved to be punished, but without ever coming out and demanding the spanking she wanted. Charlotte –

"They never took the hint, although I know Rory would have done, or you. I suppose most men just aren't natural spankers, or maybe they'd like to but can't believe I'd really want it. I used to long to be spanked, and I'd think about it all the time. Then when I did get it I could barely cope with what happened. It was my own Godfather, 'Uncle' Colin, the dirty old bastard! Don't get me wrong, he'd always been really good to me, nothing out of order, not ever. It was me who suggested it."

"You asked your Godfather for a spanking!?"

Not really asked, it wasn't like that. I was drinking with a group of friends, mostly boys, and he came past. I suppose he thought they were trying to get me drunk and I'd end up getting gang-banged or something, but we used to drink together all the time and they never took advantage. Well, not beyond asking for a flash of my tits anyway."

"Which you gave them?"

"Yes. Why not?"

"No reason at all. So what happened?"

"Uncle Colin insisted on giving me a lift home. I could have said no, but otherwise I was going to have to walk, and I was used to doing as he told me. So I got into his car, and it must have been obvious that I was a bit drunk, because he was laughing, and then he said it, these exact words – 'It's a good job you don't get spanked, Miss Charlotte'. That was it, just a joke really, but it was as if I'd had an electric shock, and the words were out of my mouth before I could stop myself – 'Oh yeah, and I suppose you'd be the one to do it, would you?'. That was it, and he just laughed, but when I got home I was so wet and horny that I had to go up and play with myself in my room before tea. I'd never felt so guilty afterwards, because I'd been imagining how it would have been if he'd stopped the car and done it, with me over his knee on the back seat with my jeans and knickers down, or made to bend over the bonnet with my bum stuck out, even done in front of my friends."

"That's a favourite of yours, isn't it?"

"Yes, and that's why."

I have a picture, taken after a party, of Charlotte bent over the bonnet of my old Rover 214 in a car park somewhere in West London. Her hands are on the bonnet, her feet braced well apart, her pleated rubber skirt turned up and her rubber panties stretched taut between her high-heeled ankle boots. She is looking back at the camera, her face set in a sleepy, happy smile, more than happy to be showing off every rude detail of her rear view, her red bottom, the tight dimple of her anus and her distinctly wet pussy. It wasn't the only time, and I'd always wondered why she was so keen on that particular pose. Back to Charlotte –

"But he didn't actually spank you?"

"Not that time, but I think after that we both knew it was going to happen. He must have picked up on something, the way I reacted probably, because after that it became a sort of running joke between us, always in private. He'd threaten and I'd tease, but I don't think he'd have gone through with it if I hadn't kept pushing him."

"What did you do?"

"I kept misbehaving, really silly things like spilling coffee, even breaking stuff. I couldn't ask him, but I just wanted it so badly, just for him to take me across his knee and smack my bottom for me, that was all, no sex, just a spanking. I was sure he wanted to, and I was hoping that if I made him angry he'd do it for real. I suppose I knew it would turn him on, but it was all really mixed up in my head and I didn't care as long as I got that spanking. I remember the day. I told him I'd been shoplifting, which I hadn't, then admitted it was a lie, and he realised what I was after, and I suppose he couldn't resist."

"I can imagine. I'd have done it, I think. After all, you were a grown girl and you're not even his real niece."

"Exactly, so why not? I suppose that was what was going through his head, because he could see the state I was in, and then he just said it – 'I suppose I better give you that spanking then'. I think I just nodded, and after that he didn't even hesitate. He must be a spanker at heart, and maybe he'd wanted to do it for a long time. I don't know, but he knew what he was doing, and how to deal with me and not take any nonsense, over his knee, a quick rub to my bottom through my skirt, my skirt turned up and my knickers taken down, and smack, smack, smack, right on my bare bum. Oh it felt nice, even nicer than I'd imagined it or when I used to spank myself and imagine a man doing it. I didn't care who it was, I just wanted it to carry on, and before I even knew what I was doing I was pushing my bum up."

"That doesn't surprise me."

"It's just how I react."

"You really like spanking, don't you? I mean actually being spanked. So many girls like the anticipation and the after effects but not the actual spanking."

"I don't get that at all, but then I do have a high pain threshold."

"So I notice. Carry on."

53

"I was over his knee, pushing my bum up and lost in this lovely feeling. I wanted it to go on for ever, just lying there all bare and warm. I felt so safe, as if by spanking me he was protecting me in some way. That was the first time I'd ever known how it feels to be mastered, as well as spanked. He smacked me so hard too, and for so long, until my bum was ablaze and I was dizzy with it. I suppose he didn't want the experience to be over, and nor did I, but in the end he couldn't stop himself from getting horny with me. He started to touch my bum between smacks and to feel between my legs. I couldn't stop him. I couldn't stop myself, and when he finally stopped and let me down on the floor I was clinging to him and shaking. He pulled out his cock and tried to put it in my mouth, pushing me down. I tried to stop myself, but I couldn't."

"So you sucked him off?"

"More than that. I let him put it in my mouth, trying to make excuses to myself, like that it was only fair when I'd got him so horny, and he was already rock hard. But I wanted him inside me and I knew I was going to do it unless he came really quickly, so I was sucking like anything, but he wouldn't do it and in the end I just gave in and sat on his lap, taking his cock and putting it up me. He put his hands on my bum, squeezing my cheeks and spanking me while I rode his cock and telling me what a naughty girl I was and how badly I'd needed spanking. I suppose the truth is that I'd had it coming for years."

Bagpipes and Bondage – Mikki Lyons

We first met Mikki when she was just starting out on the

fetish scene, nineteen years old and as eager as she was innocent. She was also highly desirable, pert, pretty and a natural exhibitionist with plenty to show off, legs that seemed to last for ever, long golden hair and a bottom to die for. My clearest memory of her from those early days comes from one of The Firm's famous boat parties, a Thames cruise with a difference. Mikki was in a classic fetish outfit, a black pvc body that left all the important bits bare, fishnet tights and outrageous heels. The way the fishnet hugged the cheeks of her bottom was heart-stopping, displaying her curves to perfection. As she climbed the companionway in front of me I remember marvelling that a girl so slim could carry such gloriously full, meaty cheeks and that human flesh could be so buoyant, and so spankable.

By then she was already a regular playmate, and I'd had my hands on those divine cheeks many a time, and yet when it came to the interview – held in the boardroom of one of the City's most prestigious institutions – neither of us could remember the details of the first occasion. Mikki –

"It must have been at the Whiplash Market, I think, or maybe at one of your parties, where it just seemed to be *de rigueur*."
"I wasn't the first though?"
"Maybe the fifth, or the sixth. Not that I'd have minded, and anyway, everyone knew that if you went to one of the Birches' parties you'd end up getting spanked."
"We endeavour to give satisfaction."

Mikki's not the first girl to remark that being spanked by me seemed an inevitable fate, but then our parties were carefully designed to ensure that everybody got theirs. After all, it would be the height of bad manners to leave anybody out. The Whiplash Market, meanwhile, would have meant her spanking was in a fairly public setting, which I ought to remember but don't, so it was probably a party, at which up to a dozen girls might get spanked, sometimes simultaneously. In any case, I wasn't her first. That came before she got involved with the fetish scene, because she is one of those determined young women who knows what she wants and usually gets it without too much delay. Mikki –

"I must have been quite young. It wasn't long after I'd left school, I think. When the hell would it have been? Hang on, I'm running through my list of boyfriends, but none of them were kinky. I tried to lure them into things, but all they ever seemed to want was straight sex."

"With you offering kinky sex? I find that hard to believe!"

"I think most men are just sexually dull, the sausage and mash variety, fine if you're starving hungry but you quickly tire of it if you have it every day. One wants to sample rare delicacies and exotic fruits as well as the staples. They just find the whole thing uncomfortable."

"Sex or kinky sex?"

"Kinky sex. It's like asking them to act. Spanking a girl needs some imagination, and some confidence. Social taboos kick in too. You'd be amazed how many men think they're rebels but really toe the line. Many are simply too lazy or more focussed on their own immediate pleasure. It's a shame, because the natural highs that they miss out on are off the scale, and all it needs is a bit of give and take."

"But you got it in the end?"

"Yes. My first time. In my year off I went on a trip to Australia, on my own. On my last evening, after an awful lot of wine I got talking about sex to a man who played the bagpipes."

"Seriously? Not the guitar, or the saxophone maybe?"

"No, the bagpipes. He was attractive, and I decided to be blatantly honest and tell him exactly what I wanted, to be put in bondage and given a good beating. To my amazement he said it was fantastic as he was into the same thing. We were already at his place by then, and we'd been in the Jacuzzi together, so it was going to happen. He ordered me to go upstairs, and lie straddled on the bed to wait for him. My adrenaline was pumping and I remember thinking – 'At last!'."

"You'd asked to be tied up and spanked, specifically?"

"More or less, but it didn't work out that way. He came upstairs and slapped me around the face so hard I lost an earring. I was sure that wasn't right, but I was a novice and so I thought – 'okay'. But he kept going for my face, even when I offered him my bum. Okay, he did slap it a bit, but he obviously hadn't got a clue, so I made my excuses and left."

"Not a very successful first spanking. What happened next?"

"It didn't put me off because I knew there must be someone competent. I was determined the next time it would be right. For me, that is, and I don't want it to seem that what happened lacked consent. What it lacked was sensuality, and that's crucial."

"So you came back to London?"

"Yes. I wanted to explore and I went out a lot. After a while a friend introduced me to Robin, who was setting up Club Whiplash at the time. He gave me a flyer. I went, my courage screwed up, expecting to see what it was like and leave after five minutes. I stayed all night. My eyes were opened to a whole new world of wonderful, genuine people, erotic adventurers like myself."

The first part of Mikki's interview had left me wondering just how many girls with spanking fantasies had been put off by incompetent men, because I felt she'd been extraordinarily brave to continue her search after her first experience. Not that it had actually been dangerous, but as she had said it had lacked sensuality and completely failed to meet her expectations. It also seemed a shame not to record a better example –

"Can you remember who gave you your first satisfying spanking?"
"John, a playmate I had around about the time I met you. He was sub, mainly, and introduced me to the joys of topping. I recall the first time I visited him. There was lots of equipment at his apartment, and implements displayed about the place. I enquired what his cleaner made of the display – he claimed she just didn't it pay any attention. He had hooks around the door frames, and after we'd been out to dinner one evening he strung me up with yellow ribbons, standing in a doorway, with my arms and legs braced apart. I was in a party frock, because we'd been out to dinner, and he pulled it right up over my chest and then took my knickers down to get me bare. It was all very gentle, and he spanked me at first by hand and proceeded to work his way through various implements, but he was good at it, and I was tied up and being beaten by a man. Perfect. I thanked him sometime later by tying him up by the ankles and shaving his head but that's another story !"

Going Down the Pub – Lavinia Martins

Lavinia has vivid memories of her first spanking and that's

no surprise. It was done in public. That's not something I would advocate, of course, but that's what happened and the story should be told as it was.

It was Penny who first met Lavinia, at a girls only party dedicated to fetish, domination and submission. They were the only two real spanking enthusiasts there, and took turns over each other's knees in the kitchen before being caught by the others, taken into the main room and strung up from a ring in the ceiling with their wrists in cuffs and their toes only just touching the floor. Both had their clothing interfered with, leaving them face to face with their near-naked bodies touching as they were whipped by the other girls, a great way to kick off a new friendship.

Like us, Lavinia and her boyfriend, another Peter, were new to the fetish scene at the time but had been together for a while. He was very much into the psychology of domination and submission, and also loved to shock. Lavinia –

"Peter is perfect for me, because I love to make an exhibition of myself but I'm really too shy. He just doesn't care. He'll even go to work in rubber trousers, more to be defiant than because he gets a kick out of it, so he's perfect to bring me out of myself."

"And he introduced you to spanking?"

"No. Spanking was my thing. It's just the best way to be an exhibitionist, so other people don't realise you're doing it on purpose. I even remember how it started. I love pin-up art, especially when a girl's showing her bum by accident and she's been seen. Sometimes the girls get spanked – they were really into it in the 50s – and I love the way they're being made to show their bare bums and can't do a thing about it, and of course, it's not their fault, because they're being spanked, and who volunteers to get spanked!?"

59

"I can think of plenty, but yes, I understand. So for you it's all about showing off?"

"At first, yes, mainly having to go bare in front of lots and lots of people. I always used to imagine it on the beach at first, with me losing my bikini in the sea and ending up in the nude with everyone looking. Or there's that poster where a dog's got hold of a girl's knickers and pulled them down, or is it a chimpanzee? Anyway, her bum's bare and everybody's looking. I'd love something like that to happen to me, but it has to be something I can't do anything about, which is why spanking's so perfect."

"And you told Peter?"

"Of course. He used to love to hear my fantasies, and to try to make them real. We were on the Heath once and he pinned me down and took off my knickers under my skirt and made me walk all the way back to the flat like that. It was windy, and one unlucky gust and I'd have been showing it all! The only trouble there was that if somebody had seen they'd just have thought I was going bare for the fun of it. They wouldn't know I'd had my knickers stripped off."

"But he didn't spank you?"

"That was later, but we had been on the Heath, to the Spaniard's, where we'd had quite a lot to drink, then to another pub, which had better remain nameless. There's a big cruising ground up there, and Peter had been teasing me by threatening to make me offer blow jobs to some of the gay guys we'd seen. I wanted to get him back, and maybe egg him into doing something rude with me, but I did not expect what he did. We'd just sat down, side by side on a bench in the beer garden, which looks out over the car park. There was this young guy in tight shorts, obviously up for it, maybe for hire, so when Peter

60

suggested I go down and proposition him I came back quick as a flash, telling him I'd go over, but that I'd tell the guy my boyfriend had a secret fantasy about sucking another man's cock and how much would it be. The next moment I was over Peter's knee, with my bum stuck right up and my knickers showing. It was such a shock, and so good I nearly fainted, I swear. And then he'd started to spank me, really hard, calling me a cheeky little slut and everything. I couldn't have stopped him if I'd wanted to, and if he'd pulled my knickers down I'd have come, I swear. Of course he couldn't, but I wish he had. Imagine, bare bum in a beer garden with all those people staring at me! Yum."

"So there were other people there?"

"Oh yes. I remember one old guy sitting on his own with a pint while he read the paper, and a couple, and I think one other single guy, maybe more. They all got a good eyeful of my knickers, and, do you know, not one of them said anything. It was all over in a few seconds anyway, and Peter made me drink up and we left before anything could happen. I made him take me in the woods and sucked his cock to say thank you, and all the while I was sucking I couldn't stop thinking of how I'd been spanked, over and over. I was playing with myself too, and that was the best orgasm of my life, I swear. That was my first, and I know I've done loads more since then, but I think it's still the best."

Age and Authority – Lauren Taylor

Lauren is a bubbly, vivacious young woman with a mop of black curls and an hourglass figure; breasts so large that each makes a full handful for any man lucky enough to get

61

hold of them, a tiny waist and a full, heavy bottom. The first time I met her she was dressed as a schoolgirl, her hair in bunches, her big breasts straining out the front of her blouse. When I complimented her on her look she immediately showed me her knickers, flipping up the back of her red tartan school skirt. They were white, full cut and tight across her big cheeks. I got to pull them down later that same evening, for an OTK spanking while Penny waited impatiently for her own turn, not to be spanked, but to spank Lauren.

Even to see her working in her smart city suit it's hard not to think sex and there's nothing she likes better than a good spanking, firm but not too hard and delivered while she brings herself to orgasm across a man's knees, preferably an older man, because the fantasies running through her head as she does it will be all to do with discipline. That's her thing, to imagine that she's being punished by a much older man, a man with authority over her, what she calls a spanking Daddy. This is not intended to be a study of the psychology of spanking, so rather than attempting an analysis of the Electra Complex I shall simply let Lauren speak for herself –

"One man who spanked me took it for granted that I'd been a Daddy's girl and that he was a substitute, but that's almost opposite to the truth. My father was almost never there, and when he was he never paid much attention to me. I wanted that attention, but I did not want to be spanked! That came later, after I found out how nice it felt to have a warm bum."

"And who gave you one?"

"Mr Fielding."

"David Fielding, who you were with when we met?"

"Yes, but I always like to think of my spankers as Mister. Being spanked by some guy called Dave or Pete just isn't the same thing ... is it, Mr Birch?"

"Fair enough. We'll come back to that, but I thought you'd been into it for years. You certainly always seemed to know what you wanted."

"I know what I like, and that's being spanked. What's to learn?"

"Not a great deal, I suppose, when you're on the receiving end. Dishing it out is another matter."

"Another good reason for going for older men. They're more experienced, usually anyway, and they're more patient with me."

"You like a long spanking, don't you?"

"Yes. I hate it when somebody isn't really into it and just wants to get it over so he can have sex. You know, sex sex. Older men are usually more patient, and more grateful."

"But what you really like is the idea of an authority figure?"

"Yes."

"Describe your ideal man."

"He'd be over fifty. Grey-haired. Stern. In a suit. Smart ... or maybe not so smart. Sometimes I like it a bit pervy."

"Tall?"

"Yes, but that's not so important. Everybody's taller than me."

"Okay, I can see David's appeal. I remember him saying that it was you who made the first move. Is that true?"

"I picked him up, yes, at a conference. I think he thought I was taking the piss, at first."

"But it was him who introduced spanking into your relationship?"

"Yes. That first night. He's like you. If there's no spanking he's not interested."

"So what happened?"

"Like I said, he seemed a bit doubtful at first and he was quite reserved, but that only encouraged me. I don't think we'd been talking more than a few minutes when he first said I was naughty. I thought he meant naughty as in sexy, not as in a bad girl who needs a spanking, and I really had no idea that's what he was after until we went up to his room."

"You'd already decided to have sex with him?"

"I didn't want to sleep alone, and he appealed to me."

"So you let him take you to his room. Where was this?"

"Birmingham. The conference was at a big hotel. Yes, we went up to his room. I asked him if he'd like me to strip for him, as I'm quite good, but he said I was a very naughty girl for suggesting it and that I deserved a spanking."

"So you got it?"

"I though he was joking at first, but he sat down on the bed and told me to get across his lap in this really firm voice. It was his voice that did it. I felt as if I'd melted and I just couldn't stop myself. I did ask him not to do it hard though, and I was scared because I thought it would hurt."

"Didn't it?"

"Not at first. He knew how to handle me, you see, and like I said, experience counts. Now that I've been given it hard on cold skin I think I'd have stopped him if he'd done that, but he was nice about it, smacking my cheeks with his cupped hand and feeling me up a lot, getting really pervy over my bum, which I liked. It felt really dirty."

"Were you bare?"

"Not at first. He seemed content with feeling me through my skirt, and it was more feeling than spanking, but there was enough, and I'd begun to get that lovely warm feeling before he even started to pull my up skirt."

"You were in a business suit?"

"Yes, and so was he. He looked so stern, like an old-fashioned headmaster or the boss of a firm or something. That was part of the thrill. I love men in suits, much more than fetish gear."

"So he turned your skirt up?"

"Yes. He told me I was a naughty girl because I was obviously enjoying myself, and that he'd have to teach me a lesson by taking my knickers down. He took ages though, pulling my skirt right up around my waist and having a good feel of my bum through my knickers before he pulled them down, spanking me too, and telling me how naughty I was and how red my bum was."

"So how did you feel? Embarrassed?"

"Not really. Maybe a bit, but it was mainly just fun, a new game, and the warm feeling was lovely. Once my knickers were down he started to do it quite hard, but I was so horny I didn't mind. I wanted to play with myself, to make myself come."

"And did you?"

"Yes. I couldn't stop myself. You know I like to play with myself while I'm spanked."

"How did he react?"

"He pretended to be furious, telling me I was a dirty slut and all sorts, spanking harder as well, but the harder he spanked the worse I got, sticking my bum right up and trying to show him what I was doing and everything. I could feel his cock too and I knew it would be going in me, but he didn't stop spanking until I'd come. That was special."

"I can imagine. So that was your first spanking, but you always say you like to feel you're being punished?"

"He liked me to feel I was being punished, and it works for me. Most of what I'm into comes from him, but it was like he'd keyed in to something inside me. I never knew I needed to feel I was being punished before, and it was him who made me call him Mr Fielding. Really I think he'd rather have a girl who didn't like it quite so much, but he's a great spanking Daddy, and I can think of somebody else who is too, Mr Birch."

After that there was only one thing to do. Spank her myself.

Vicious – Julie Bourne

Julie is, quite simply, the dirtiest girl I've ever come across. When I first met her we'd already been involved with the fetish scene for five years and there was very little I hadn't seen or done. She still managed to shock me, not so much for what she'd done – which is best left to the imagination even in this book – but for the casual way in which she described it to me within five minutes of meeting. Admittedly she knew who I was and what I was into, and we were on our way to film her wallowing in the mud as a human pig, but I was still taken aback. The film crew were more taken aback still. Julie is tiny, scarcely five feet tall and petite, with ginger hair and huge, pale grey eyes. She looks as if butter wouldn't melt in her mouth, so innocent that at the beginning of the shoot they were convinced that she must have been coerced if not actually forced into taking part. On the way out to the location she was explaining that she preferred men with small cocks because they could sodomise her more easily, which disabused them of any false notions of her innocence, while by the end of the day they seemed positively alarmed. By then I'd spanked her, warming her bottom across my knee to get her in the mood for her session in the mud wallow. She was already naked, and she stayed that way, walking back to the cars in nothing but a towel, and that so short it left the cheeks of her red, mud-smeared bottom peeping out from underneath as she walked.

We'd been introduced by a mutual friend when I was looking for a girl wanton enough and kinky enough to do the piggy-girl piece, which is quite a story in itself. As it was I had several volunteers, but Julie got in first with what I soon learnt was typical enthusiasm. She brought the same attitude to everything, plunging into the club and party scene with boundless exuberance. A night in bed with her was said to be like trying to have sex with a wild cat, not that I'd know. Sadly she was only in London a few months before she moved away, but I did manage to get hold of the story of her first spanking, which is every bit as wild as I might have expected. Julie –

"He was a man I met at college. I was doing art and design and he was a part-time tutor. He fancied me right from the start and we ended up in bed. I thought he was a bit normal, but he could fuck hard, only when I started to scratch he'd stop. He kept doing that, and telling me to stop it, but I scratch. I can't help it, when someone's got his cock inside me. He didn't seem to think of tying me up, or turning me over, at first. I really thought he was going to walk out on me, and I was getting pretty pissed off. Then all of a sudden he pulls out, grabs me and twists my arm behind my back, forcing me face down on the bed. I thought he was going to put it up my bum, but instead he starts to spank me, calling me a vicious little bitch as he lays into my bum, really hard. I was furious, calling him a bastard and telling him to get off me, until I realised just how horny it was. My bum

67

was so hot and I could feel his stiff cock against my leg as he spanked me. He started to rub it on me and I knew he was getting off. I thought I knew where it was going too, up my bum, but he just carried on spanking and rubbing on my leg, never once saying a word, until I felt it get hot and wet on my cheeks. He'd spunked on my bottom."

It's all too easy to imagine her, stark naked, her legs kicking and her copper-coloured hair flying, her pale skin making the fiery red of her smacked bottom stand out more vividly even than normal, and the red in turn spattered with the white of her lover's come. With anybody but Julie I'd be worried about the issue of consent, and it was certainly a rough way to start. Yet she not only enjoyed it but took to it with all her boundless enthusiasm, so that, by the time I met her, when she was just out of that same college, she'd come to regard being spanked as an essential part of foreplay. After the filming she told me that had I not reddened her bottom for her she would have felt insulted.

Sapphic Scotland – Rosie MacIntyre

When I interviewed Rosie we were both sure that we must have met each other and possibly even played together during the 90s, but neither of us could remember for certain. They were heady days for both of us, with clubs and parties every week, and it was by no means unusual to play with a dozen people over the course of an evening, so perhaps it's not surprising that I can't recall every incident. I do remember when we met again after both of us had been taking a break from the scene. It was at Night of the Cane and I had been giving a demonstration of punishment techniques with Leia-Ann Woods. Some time later two young dominas I'd not met before came up to me and asked

68

if I could repeat part of my demonstration for their benefit. Leia-Ann had escaped and there was nobody else suitable nearby, so I offered to do as they asked if they could provide a suitable bottom as a target. My hope was that one or other of them would volunteer, preferably both, as there are few things I like better than spanking and caning a sexually dominant woman.

That was not to be, but one of them immediately went off to find a volunteer and returned a few minutes later with a pretty, dark-haired girl who they introduced to me as Rosie. She looked somewhat bemused and didn't seem to be at all sure what was going on, but both her friends assured me it was all right as they bent her over a whipping stool and stripped her bottom for the cane. I was a little hesitant, but went ahead with my demonstration, spanking her first to warm her bottom and then applying six firm strokes of the cane to create the five-bar gate effect they had wanted to see, with the last stroke placed diagonally across the others. To my delight, and some relief, Rosie thoroughly enjoyed the experience. Since then we've played on several occasions, and had I known how experienced she was, and that she likes it rough, I wouldn't have been so hesitant. Rosie –

"You didn't really do it hard enough. Scarlett had told me I was going to get a good thrashing, you see, and when I didn't I felt a bit cheated."

"I do apologise, but you looked bemused."

"Only because I didn't know what was going on. One minute I'm having a quiet drink and the next I'm being dragged away for a beating from a man I've never met."

"Fair enough. I hope I've made up for it since?"

"Oh yes, but oddly enough it was a bit like that for my first spanking too."

"So have you always liked it hard?"

"I've always liked it quite hard, not too hard, but hard enough to hurt. That's the whole idea, isn't it?"

"Tastes vary."

They do, but Rosie is a classic masochist, enjoying the pain for its own sake as well as all the trappings of spanking fantasy, especially the idea of being punished. She also switches, dishing it out with an effective skill born of her own experience of being on the receiving end. That, coupled with a wry and distinctly wicked sense of humour, makes her an excellent playmate and just the person to get a kinky party off the ground, and to keep it going. Not that you'd guess, as her wholesome looks and quiet dress sense suggest that she's more likely to be using cane to make wickerwork baskets than to punish naughty boys. She does both, nowadays, but for many years she was purely lesbian and her favourite thrill is still to be punished by another woman, as she was for her first ever spanking experience. Rosie –

"Anyway, you wanted to ask me about my first spanking. It was with a woman I corrupted."

"You corrupted her?"

"Oh, yes. It was the only way I was going to get what I wanted. This was in the early 90s, on the west coast of Scotland. We didn't have the internet, and the only clubs were hundreds of miles away in London. I didn't even know about them."

"But you knew you wanted to be spanked?"

"Beaten. I always thought of it as beaten. Yes, always."

"And what happened?"

"I was studying in Oban. We used to go to a pub, which I'd better not name, but it was halfway up the hill at the back of the town. It was a popular student pub and they had lesbian evenings, which was pretty daring thereabouts, even in the 90s. It all took place in a hut at the back so we wouldn't scare the locals."

"A hut?"

"It was habitable. It had its own bar. Mostly it was all talk and no action, but one evening I got talking to a woman who turned out to be a complete rogue. She was called Maria and she was an Irish Catholic, but really fiery and rebellious, wicked too. She was telling me how she and her friends used to watch each other pee but never dared admit to getting off on what they could see. I was feeling frustrated and horny, and the more she talked the worse I got. I didn't know if she'd be up for beating me, but I thought if she was pervy enough to enjoy watching her friends pee she might like to beat me, or at least be prepared to give it a go. I wanted to make something happen, so I sat on her lap and told her a story about a naughty girl who had to be sent to the headmistress and got the strap."

"Is that one of your favourite fantasies?"

"Yes, especially the idea of feeling that there's no way out, but it went with what we'd been talking about too, girls being naughty, and I really wanted to provoke her into beating me. Like I said, I'd always wanted it and at last it looked as if I'd met somebody who might do it. Not that I got it, not that first night."

"That's a shame."

"It was still a good night. The best I'd had. We went back to her flat and had rough sex, but there was nothing SM about it."

"Hang on. A lot of people would say that rough sex is SM, or at least close to it. What did you actually do?"

"Oh, she held me by my hair to make me lick her out, and she kept climbing on top of me to rub herself on my legs and belly, and she sat on my face to make me lick her like that."

71

"A bit of domination and submission at the very least. I'm surprised she didn't spank you. I would have done."

"Obviously, but you're a complete pervert. She just wanted to be in charge. There was a really embarrassing incident though. We were very loud, and we were at it nearly all night. Her grown-up son came in the next morning when we were still in bed and complained."

"Embarrassing is about right! So no spanking that night, but she was the first to spank you?"

"Yes. We talked the next day, and I couldn't keep it inside me any more, so I told her I wanted to be beaten. She was a bit taken aback and I had to explain what I meant, which was nearly as embarrassing as being caught by her son, but a major turn-on too."

"And she agreed to do it?"

"Yes, once I'd managed to convince her I really wanted it, and she did like being rough with me after all. We couldn't really do it at her house though, because it was bound to be even noisier than before, and I was in student digs, which was worse."

"Hang on, she obviously wasn't a student if she had her own house and a grown-up son, so …"

"Never you mind what she was, Peter Birch."

"Oh, I see. Anyway, carry on."

"We agreed to meet up at a friend's house outside the town, which was much more discreet. We weren't, because we were so turned on we were snogging in the back of the cab on the way. I remember going into the house, and being flattered by how much effort she'd put in for me, with a big room lit by tea lights, and the little whip she'd bought to use on me, just a toy really, one of those little riding whips with a leather hand at the end. She must have got it from the

72

local equestrian centre. She didn't really know what she was doing, but she was keen to oblige, giving me orders right from the start. I was keen too, and I'd bought myself a lacy black underwear set which I thought she might like. She did, because when she made me strip she said to leave my stockings and suspender belt on and that she would remove my knickers and camisole top. That was amazing, standing there are she turned my top up to feel my breasts then pulled my knickers down and left me standing like that, knowing I was going to be beaten. I wanted it so badly, and I could feel all those years of frustration bubbling up inside me, but I was still really nervous, shaking and scared of the pain. Like I said, the whip was really just a toy, but I was sure it would hurt like anything. She made me put my hands on my head and she came round behind me, talking to me and telling me what a bad girl I'd been and using the end of the tip to stroke my flesh, my bottom, but mainly my breasts, until my nipples were so hard they ached. I kept thinking she was going to hit me. My trembling was getting worse and worse, and the longer she held off the more scared I was getting, but in the end she barely touched me, just using the tip to smack my bottom a few times and then twisting her hand in my hair to force me down onto my knee for a lick. That part was great, but I'd wanted to be beaten properly first and she seemed to think it ought to be just a bit titillating. I wanted more, but I didn't want to upset her, so I didn't say anything but just put up with it. It was really frustrating, but it was a good night, and we were at it all night, sex anyway. Oh, and that night made us notorious in Oban, which is really small, mainly because we'd been snogging in the cab. Soon all the drivers knew, and that meant everybody knew, but only that we were lesbians, not the juicy details, never mind what I'd have liked to have happened."

"So it never really got weird enough for you?"

"No. I didn't get that until I came to London the year after. I knew exactly what I wanted and joined up with a lesbian SM group straight away. That was when all the business with Spanner* was going on, so I'd soon met other people, and for the first time in my life men I felt attracted to. I joined in the marches, and there was a cabaret afterwards with lots of girls in school uniform. I asked if I could join in and they let me, but when I threw and apple and hit the head girl she put me over her knee and beat me really hard. Why are you laughing?"

"Because I organised the cabaret and the woman who spanked you was my wife, Penny. We always wondered who the girl who threw the apple was, and now I know. I knew I'd met you some time around then!"

* The Spanner Case, which involved the prosecution of a group of gay men for consensual sadomasochistic acts. The case went all the way to the European Court, and while it ultimately failed it was important in bringing together different elements of the SM community and in sending a clear message that SMers were prepared to fight back.

Just Desserts – Sophie Blackwater

I first met, and spanked, Sophie comparatively recently, although she is now one of my favourite playmates. At the time Penny wasn't going to fetish clubs at all and I only ever made those run by The Firm, including their annual Boat Party. This is one of the highlights of the fetish calendar and takes a lot of organising. I'd volunteered to help out, which meant heavy lifting and handling freshly painted equipment. For this work I wore overalls, and by the time the boat put out on to the Thames these were smeared with paint marks, while I'd left what I'd intended to wear in the car. Everybody else was dressed in fetish finery, and my attempts to persuade potential playmates that I'd come as a janitor didn't really work. Eventually I gave up and settled down with a drink in the stern of the boat, content to watch other people, and there were some very fine sights indeed.

Perhaps finest of all was a girl in an immaculate white naval uniform, complete with peaked cap and gold insignia. The cheeks of her small, rounded bottom pushed out the seat of her uniform trousers in the most intriguing way, while she had extraordinarily long legs and straight brown hair down to the small of her back. Just to watch her walk was a delight, and before too long I'd decided that she was simply too fine to be ignored. I approached her with every expectation of the sort of look a tramp might get on walking in on a society ball, promptly followed by rejection. To my delight she was happy to play, her only stipulation being that we had to take turns. That was fine by me, and although she managed to break the zip of my overalls and leave me looking more disreputable than ever, that did nothing to dilute my pleasure as I pulled down her uniform trousers and the tiny panties beneath to treat her to a hand spanking and a session with her own suede flogger.

We talked for a while afterwards, and she proved to be one of the nicest and most sympathetic people I had ever met. She also has a wonderful enthusiasm for spanking, a strong exhibitionist streak and a love of costume and erotic display that mirrors my own tastes. One thing I especially like about her is a streak of naivety, which she has never lost for all her experience, and which is reflected in her interview. Sophie –

"My first spanking? I was tempted into it! Not that I didn't enjoy it. Well, you know that as well as anybody, but I was definitely tempted. I'd only been involved with the fetish scene a few months, and while I was having a great time it was all fem dom. That suited me, and in a way it seemed to be what was expected of me. There was no shortage of men eager to be dominated, that's for sure."

"I can imagine. But what did you want to do, at heart?"

"Be sexy. I'm an exhibitionist by nature and playing kinky is a great way to show off. That's why I'd chosen the outfit I was in that night. It was a black PVC body, very tight and with cut-outs on the chest so my breasts were bare. I had thighs boots too, and long black PVC gloves. The boys loved it, and I had men asking to lick my boots and for me to beat them and if they could be my personal slave, everything."

"This was at a fetish club?"

"Yes. I won't say which, but it was one of the big ones. I was having a great time, anyway, and trying to keep as many men happy as I could. One of them was desperate to be caned, so I took him into the dungeon. There was a lot of action going on, men and women beating each other all around, and I had to join a queue for the equipment. The man – who was called Peter, oddly enough – went to get me a drink and I was left watching this really glamorous T-girl while she beat a man over a whipping stool. Like I said, I'd only been around a few months, and while I'd bought lots of equipment I wasn't one hundred per cent confident about using it. The T-girl knew exactly what she was doing. In fact she was really showing off. I'd have been okay just watching, but she picked up on my interest and asked if I'd like a go.

Well, no, what she actually did was take one look at me and decide she wanted to spank and punish me, but we'll come back to that later."

"She sounds like somebody after my own heart. Do carry on."

"She asked if I'd like a go, then checked with the guy she was beating. He said yes too, so I gave him a couple of strokes with the cane. Then Joanna – the T-girl – stepped in and showed me the best way to stand and how to get the stroke right on target and really make it count at the same time. I remember feeling a bit put out, because I couldn't really see that there was much difference between what I'd done and what she wanted me to do. Really she was just trying to find an excuse to get her hands on me, and that did occur to me too, but she was nice and I didn't mind. She soon had to admit I'd got the knack anyway, so we carried on caning the guy together. I never did find out what his name was. Peter came back with my drink and got sent off to fetch one for Joanna, and when he came back we gave him his turn. He loved getting attention from both of us, and boy did he react! We had his pants down, and Joanna had made him brace his legs apart. He had a really big cock, and it swung back and forth as our canes hit his bum, all the time getting longer and harder. It was making me giggle, the way it was swinging, and it was turning me on to see him get so excited over being beaten. Joanna was great too, fun as well as sexy, and she kept giving me tips on how to handle him, and all the different implements."

"So you'd moved on from the cane?"

"Yes. We both had several different implements with us, different canes and riding crops, paddles and straps, and this beautiful purple suede flogger I'd just bought, and which you've met."

"My favourite. I'm beginning to envy the guy you were dealing with."

"Don't! The poor man got dumped. Well, not dumped exactly. He seemed to be able to take everything we could dish out, but eventually we decided we needed a break, and there were other people waiting to use the whipping stool. So we sat down and talked, with Peter curled on the floor at my feet, rubbing his face on my boots. Joanna started explaining to me about how men and women react to spankings, and well … I don't know … First I let her use one of her straps on my hand, just to see how it felt, and then on my bum to feel the difference, and before I really knew it I was the one over the whipping stool! That's what changed it from just sort of techie stuff to the real thing. You can imagine it, can't you? Over the same whipping stool I'd just used to beat a man, in front of everybody, him included, having my bottom smacked! I felt so naughty, as if I was really being punished, and so … so wrong in a way, as if I'd been brought down from on high. I was thinking what they could all see, and all the men who'd been admiring me, worshipping me, and there I was with my bum stuck up in the air, being spanked and whipped!

"Joanna was brilliant. She kept checking to see I was all right, and she took it really slowly, paying lots of attention to my neck and back as well as my bum, with her hands and the whip too. That was something else that really got to me, being beaten with my own whip. And the way I was showing off, because if I'd been showing off before now I was really exposed. It was different too, more vulnerable, just having my breasts showing, even though they'd been bare all night. This was different. And then Joanna undid my

78

body suit. She did ask, but the way she did it was really firm. Her fingers were on the buttons between my legs, right over my pussy, and she leant down and whispered in my ear – 'I think we'd better have you bare, don't you?'. That's what she said, I think. I couldn't say no, but I couldn't say yes either, not when it meant having my bare bum put on show in front of all those people, men who'd been worshipping my boots just minutes before, and other women too, other dominant women. Joanna knew just what to do. She waited a few seconds in case I couldn't handle it, and maybe to let what was about to happen to me build up in my head. Then she'd popped the buttons and lifted up the back of my body suit.

"Suddenly I was showing everything, and because I'm slim I do mean everything. All those people were watching, and it wasn't even that dark in there. The front bit had fallen down too, so my pussy was bare, and my bottom hole, and I was thinking how I'd look from behind as Joanna went back to beating me, using my own flogger on my bare bum. Now I really felt I was getting my just desserts, for being such a little show-off and for dominating all those men. And I understood what Joanna had been talking about, the way the beating made my bottom warm and got me feeling I was ready for sex, and what it did in my head, those lovely feelings of wanting to be completely exposed for everybody and to please the person who's beating me, who's punishing me. I knew why Peter hadn't wanted it to stop as well, because I felt I wanted it to go on for ever. It was such a high, and it's just as well it was Joanna and she looked after me, because if it had been somebody less considerate I think I'd have ended up a real mess and

79

just lapped it up, but maybe regretted it later. She did cane me though, six hard strokes at the very end, far harder than I could ever take cold but even that was just lovely. I was stroking my bum when she finally let me up, to feel the heat in my flesh and the marks from the cane. It felt so good, I couldn't not come. So when she came to give me a cuddle and kiss my bottom better I suggested she take me into a private corner where I could come while I gave her what it really looks like you could do with at this moment!"

After a brief intermission we resumed Sophie's interview.

"I know you're very much into fetish and exhibitionism, but domestic spanking? What was your first experience of being OTK?"

"I'm not sure. It may even have been when we met on the boat."

"No. You were over a whipping stool and then up against a ... bulkhead I think they're called. The first time I actually put you across my knee would have been at one of Ishmael's Christmas parties when I was playing Santa."

"Oh yes! I remember. I was your elf. Maybe that was my first over the knee spanking, I'm not sure. It was lovely though, to have Santa take down my panties and spank me in front of everybody. Somebody was taking photos too, weren't they?"

"Yes. I've got copies. Not that I really need them. I remember exactly how it was. You were in a red PVC dress with a flared skirt trimmed with white fluff, bright red stack heels that seemed to make your legs go on for ever. The skirt was so short you could hardly avoid showing your knickers, which were white cotton ..."

"My school panties."

"… and hugged your bottom so nicely it was almost a shame to pull them down, almost."

"You did though, didn't you, in front of about twenty people!? And you pulled the front of my dress down, which was completely unnecessary!"

"Oh, I don't know. Doesn't having your breasts bare add to your feelings when you're spanked, mainly because it isn't actually necessary in order to punish you?"

"I suppose so. That must have been my first trip over a man's knee then, knickers down and tits out over Santa's knee at a Christmas party! Only it wasn't, because if we'd met that must have been the Christmas after the Boat Party, and I had a wonderful experience earlier that year. It was in a library, where my friend Charles is in charge. He has the keys, and he took me back one evening after it was closed. He gave me a lovely OTK spanking and he spanked my pussy too, which really took me by surprise and isn't something I'd let most men do. Charles did, and he was so good he brought me off like that. Yes, that would be my first experience OTK. How could I forget!"

Taken in Hand – Mia Jay

I was introduced to Mia as a friend of Sophie's. I'd been asked to take the photographs for a flyer to promote a fetish party with a French revolution theme. The party was to be called Marat Sade and the brief was to create a picture of de Sade seated in his cell in the Bastille, quill pen in hand as he pondered on perverse fantasies. The perverse fantasies were to be depicted as three girls who would be doing lewd things to each other. They were to be half dressed and half visible,

81

as if they were the projections of de Sade's thoughts. It was quite an ambitious project, possibly too ambitious, but I like to think we did well on very limited resources. I decided to play de Sade myself and to operate the camera remotely, which left me needing three girls to model as the lewd ghosts of his imagination.

The three girls who eventually volunteered deserve medals for what they put up with, especially Mia, who I'd never met and had no idea what was expected of her. De Sade's "cell" was an alcove in the basement of a London pub and came with genuine slime-encrusted walls, thirty-degree heat and frequent visits from curious bar staff. Nevertheless, Mia, Sophie and Julie cheerfully stripped down and dressed up again in the curious outfits I'd thrown together for the piece. These were a combination of Victorian underwear, worn *déshabillée*, with Tricoleur accessories, which might not have been historically accurate for revolutionary France but might well have sprung from de Sade's foetid imagination.

I was deeply impressed by the girls' professionalism, although perhaps determination would be a better word as they weren't getting paid. Mia never complained once, even as the poses grew increasingly bizarre and intimate, right up to having her bottom kissed by Julie, who she'd met just minutes before. All three of them looked lovely, with their chemises open across bare breasts and their drawers wide to show off their bottoms and between their legs, dishevelled and wet with the sweat of passion, Mia with her blonde hair in disarray and her nipples as stiff as corks. I forget how the flyer turned out, but it will be a very long time indeed before I forget being squeezed into that tiny, baking hot space with three half-naked, giggling girls.

Another high point was playing with the three of them at the fetish event which took place in the pub upstairs after the shoot. We started by tying Julie to a cross, her arms and legs spread wide, her Victorian drawers open to display her tiny, rounded bottom for whipping. Then it was Sophie's turn, then Mia's, each girl attended to by the others while I enjoyed the view. My memory of what happened later is hazy, but I do remember both spanking and caning Mia, and being particularly impressed by how compliant she was, with a natural and very beautiful submission I found instantly arousing then and still do now. She was also both knowing and enthusiastic, so much so that I was surprised to learn from Sophie that she wasn't particularly experienced. Her first spanking had been delivered just weeks before, by Mistress Sapphira, one of the Scene's most active dominas at the time, aided and abetted by the wicked Joanna. Mia –

"I'd gone along to one of the fetish markets. All I meant to do was buy myself an outfit and maybe some accessories, because while I knew what I wanted I'd never done anything. My pet fantasy had always been to be made a plaything by another woman, a dominant woman, and I suppose that must show, because Mistress Sapphira homed in on me like a cat with a mouse. I'd only been there a few minutes when she started talking to me, at one of the bigger stalls where they sell all sorts, clothing and CP implements too. I was thinking of going to Torture Garden and I was asking for advice, mainly about what I could get away with, so I suppose it was easy for Mistress Sapphira to work out what I was into. She said she'd help me choose, but I didn't expect her to help me change."

"In the middle of the market?"

"No. The stall had a curtained-off area at the back, but it wasn't exactly well hidden. Sapphira was really matter-of-fact about me stripping off, as if it just didn't matter. Less than an hour after I'd arrived, my first ever contact with the fetish scene and I was naked in front of this really beautiful, dominant woman. Well, you know what she's like, tall and slim and just from the look on her face you know she's not going to stand any nonsense. So I ended up naked, then in a maid's outfit complete with frilly knickers and a little lace hat, then naked again, then in nothing but rubber panties and stack heels, which made me feel even more naked than with nothing on!"

"Which outfit did you buy?"

"Both, and a red rubber dress with a heart shaped cut-out at the back to show the top of my bum. I suppose my first, first spank was when I was wriggling into that, because it was really tight and Sapphira had to help me. She was trying to get it up over my hips and I suppose I was wiggling my bum a lot, and right in her face. I was about half in and half out when she smacked me, just once, as if to punish me for being a nuisance. That was all, and she did it really casually, but I couldn't get it out of my head that this wonderful woman had smacked me. I was hoping there'd be more to come."

"And there was, I take it?"

"Lots more! When we came out of the cubicle the man behind the stall suggested a red whip to go with the dress. I liked the idea, but Sapphira wasn't having it and I'll never forget what she said – 'Oh no, that's not for her, that's for me, to put across her bottom'. She bought the whip – a bright red riding crop – and told me to stick my bum out for her to test it. I'd done it before I could even think of refusing, offering her my bum to whip. The first smack was just hard enough to sting, but sent a shock right through me. I stayed as I was, hoping for more, but she just laughed and said – 'I know where we're going, my girl'. That was more than I did, but it turned out there was a little room off to one side where you could play."

"You knew you were going to be beaten though? Didn't you want to resist, even a little?"

"Why resist? Anyway, I couldn't. Sapphira took me by my hand and led me to the play room. I remember seeing the big St Andrew's Cross and thinking – 'So this is how girls are whipped' – and after that it's all just one memory running into another. Joanna was there ... do you know TV Joanna?"

"I think I know who you mean, yes."

"She was there. I think she was dungeon monitor. She knew Sapphira anyway, and I remember her looking me up and down and smiling. They put me on the cross, with my hands stretched up and my feet apart. There were leather cuffs, and I remember how helpless I felt as Sapphira fastened each one off and how Joanna kept telling me that it was going to be all right. It was Sapphira who beat me, at first. She tucked up my dress and pulled down my knickers, just as if it didn't matter at all for me to have my bum bare in what was really public."

"Were you still in your new rubber dress?"

"No. I'd changed back, to a plain blue summer dress. Once she'd got my knickers down she started to play with my bum, using the crop, not hard at all, but flicking at my cheeks and tickling underneath. After a bit she stopped to take off this long, black leather coat she was wearing and she gave the riding crop to Joanna. They shared me like that, taking turns to use the whip and their hands too, spanking me and touching me until I could barely breathe for excitement. I'd have let them do anything, and I think I was pleading with them to make me come. How dirty is that!?"

"Very, and very nice. I hope they obliged?"

"Sapphira did. They'd already pulled up my dress, and they had my knickers as far down my legs as they'd go, because I was on the cross, of course, so my body was naked from my neck to my knees."

"No bra?"

"Who needs a bra?"

"Not you, evidently (this after having two neatly formed and extremely firm tits flashed at me.) Go on."

"I was naked then, and Joanna was using the crop and her fingers on my bum and back while Sapphira came around in front of me. She started to play with my nipples, until I was so needy I was sticking my bum out for the crop and begging to be touched. She made me wait for ages, all the time looking right into my face with such a cruel expression, a lot of lust too. Finally she put a hand between my legs and began to rub me, with Joanna using the crop all the time, harder and harder until I came, and when I did, the way I screamed it's amazing the place didn't get raided by the police!"

A Teenage Secret – Rosa Abrahams

I had known about Rosa for quite a while before I met her, admiring her cheeky smile and equally cheeky bottom on the net. As she was in the Midlands and we both seemed to be plentifully supplied with playmates that is probably how matters would have stayed but for a chance meeting at the house of a mutual friend. We spoke for a while and I learned that she had a responsible job as controller for a coach company in Birmingham. It was several months later that I happened to be working in Kidderminster and decided to go on to one of the Birmingham clubs afterwards. Taking a coach seemed to be the cheapest and simplest option for travel that evening, and as the line was operated by Rosa's company I even felt a certain loyalty.

The journey proved to be a nightmare, so that I finally got to the club halfway through the evening, cold, wet and thoroughly fed up. There was Rosa, warm, dry and perched happily on her boyfriend's knee with her skirt turned up at the back and her knickers half down as he kneaded one distinctly rosy bottom cheek. He was also a friend, fortunately, and her protests that she'd gone off duty several hours before my journey began did her no good at all. I put her over my knee and took out my frustrations on her bottom, spanking her until at length the pleasure of having her wriggling on my lap with her deliciously plump, bare bottom bouncing under my hand restored my good humour. Even then she was still protesting that the spanking wasn't fair, but the wet patch on my leg told a different story.

Since then I've come to know her as great fun and a great playmate, also that while she was now bisexual she had been lesbian first and that her first ever spanking had come from another girl. It was a story I had to have. Rosa –

"It was my girlfriend's twenty-first birthday. We started the day gently, breakfast in bed, presents, cuddles. We'd been together long enough – a few months – to be comfortable with each other's rhythms, comfortable with each other's bodies. She was three years older than me, which from eighteen to twenty-one still feels like quite a big age difference and I looked up to her. She had been making her own way in the world for much longer than me."

"Were you already living together?"

"Not all the time, but I knew I'd be sleeping with her that night. The rest of the day was spent in preparation for the evening's party, cleaning the flat, getting some snacks and beers, a trip to D's for some dope and we were all set. The party was great, twenty or so women listening to music, dancing, drinking, smoking, laughing, fooling around. Even a couple of women we were friendly with from the local pub dropped in for a bit, although I think a women-only party was something of a culture shock for them. The evening wound down, people were getting tired, a bit drunk, a bit stoned, or pairing off. A lot of them were staying rather than travel across the city late at night, so we had to sort out where everyone was crashing. Eventually we went up to her room to get ready for bed. I remember her in the dim light, undressing, taking off the armour she wore for the outside world, even for a party of friends here to celebrate her birthday. I knew she didn't like her body, but she looked beautiful to me that night, her full curves and generous breasts. There was a glint of unpredictability in her eye too, a spark that simultaneously attracted and alarmed me. I knew she wasn't drunk, but she was a little stoned though, as I was too. Then it was my turn to undress and I was looking at her face as she watched me. I could see her desire, written plainly, but also something else. Our lovemaking had generally settled into a fairly predictable pattern, but I got the feeling that tonight might be a little different.

"We climbed into bed, but suddenly she jumped up to check something which she'd put down on the far side. I wondered what it was, but I didn't ask, sure I'd find out when she was ready. Then she was back in bed with me and we were in each other's arms, skin on skin, naked bodies together, a delicious sensation. She began to stroke my breasts, pinching my nipples, biting my neck too, until I'd started to moan and writhe against her. Suddenly she stopped and ordered me to get up. I wasn't sure what was going on, but she quickly made it clear, 'Up, I said. Kneel up at the head of the bed facing the wall with your hands behind your back'.

"I was too surprised to do anything other than comply. This was something new. I got into position, naked remember, and waited as she reached down the side of the bed for what she had left there earlier. When I felt something soft and cool binding my wrists I realised it was the tie of my satin dressing gown. That was such a shock, such a lovely shock that even though I was trying to be quiet I knew that whimpers of excitement were escaping my mouth and I was painfully aware that her ex-girlfriend was just the other side of the wall I was kneeling against."

"How embarrassing."

"Yes, but exciting too, and I had no idea what was going to happen next. My girlfriend was surveying me coolly, as if trying to decide what to do with me and knowing it could be anything she wanted. Then she suddenly grabbed me by the hair and the arms, pulled me away from the wall and pushed my face down into the bed. She didn't say a word all the while, but my bottom was poking up in the air so I suppose I should have guessed. I didn't, and at the first spank I squealed with surprise. 'That wasn't really very hard,' – she said, and I could hear the mockery in her voice. The next spank was less of a shock and she was right, it wasn't really that hard, the first one was just such a shock because I'd never been spanked before and I had trouble taking in why she'd want to punish me, and why it should turn her on, because it obviously did. Only as she carried on I was surprised to find that being spanked by her was really quite pleasurable. In fact I found myself getting very turned on and I couldn't help it, but it was as embarrassing as it was exciting when she paused in the spanking to slide her fingers up into my cunt and feel how wet I was.

"She started again, harder now, still with my face in the bedclothes and my bum in the air for a bit, then she pulled me back up and pushed me against the wall again. As she carried on spanking I'd begun to moan and cry out. I couldn't stop myself at all. My cunt was soaking, my bottom was sore, and I was more turned on than I'd ever been in my life. She grabbed me by the hair to hold me in position and pushed several fingers roughly into my cunt, starting to finger fuck me. I was so turned on I started to come almost immediately, and when I did it was long and hard, with her fingers pushing in and out really hard and my burning bottom pushed out onto her hand. I'd lost all awareness of what was going on around me, except for what she was doing to me and I was screaming with pleasure as I came, just not caring that we were in a house full of friends, including her ex.

"She stopped, just holding me while she let me catch my breath, but not for long. She wasn't finished with me yet. She untied my wrists, grabbed my hair and pulled my head down onto her cunt. I tasted how wet she was, and how aroused, as I started to lick. I enjoyed pleasuring her with my tongue. I always did, but this was different, special, because she'd spanked me. Usually it took a while for her to reach orgasm but not tonight. She was so turned on by what she'd done to me that it didn't seem to take any time at all until she was groaning and grinding her hips to push her cunt into my face. When she'd come we both collapsed into an exhausted sleep and in the morning our friends were teasing us about the amount of noise we'd been making, but they didn't realise what had happened, so we just laughed and grinned at each other, a secret smile for what we shared."

Bad Reputation – new friends, new spankings

IT'S NOW BEEN NEARLY two decades since Penny and I first went out on the fetish scene, and life moves on. There used to be a handful of clubs, nearly all of them in London, and everybody knew everybody else, just about. Nowadays there are dozens of clubs, all over the country, and thousands of people involved, hundreds of thousands if you include those who come out only in the virtual world. On the rare occasions we do go out we find we hardly know anybody, but that no longer matters. We were out and proud for long enough to ensure that our reputation has spread, making it easy to find new spanking playmates, many of who have never been to a fetish club at all, or if they have still much prefer to play in a comfortable, home environment, as we do ourselves. We've also been making our way in the world as authors of erotic fiction, which has proved to be another excellent source of playmates.

Alphabetical Spanking – Zoe East

I had heard about Zoe long before I met her. Guy was a friend and rival in the alphabetical spanking competition held among a group of male spankers. He used to boast about her wild antics, and that she was his Z. The aim of the alphabetical spanking game is to have spanked at least one girl whose first name began with each letter of the alphabet. Five of us were involved at the time, more or less on an even footing with our alphabets half finished or a little more. We all had plenty of As, Js, Ns and the other common letters, but it was beginning to get tricky, which was why he was particularly proud of himself to have found, and spanked, a Zoe. Naturally I had to catch up, and did so by persuading a notoriously tough Mistress whose name also begins with Z to take a few gentle pats on her bottom in return for doing things to me that I'd rather not go into.

That didn't mean I wasn't interested in Zoe, far from it, but when I finally got to meet her I found out that she much preferred to play with other women. It was Penny who spanked her first, on the day we met and in the middle of a wood, although I can't remember for the life of me what we were doing there, aside from spanking Zoe. It's a picture that remains firmly in my mind: Penny seated on a tree stump with Zoe cuddled into her, Penny fully dressed, Zoe naked but for a minuscule pair of frilly panties. Those panties had quickly been pulled down, leaving Zoe bare behind, her anus on show between her cheeks, her pussy spread across Penny's leg as they kissed. Penny spanked her like that, a gloriously rude position, as I stood and watched, wondering if Zoe was sufficiently debauched to mind me pulling out my cock to masturbate over her rear view. I decided against it, on such short acquaintance, but I did get to spank her, with Penny holding her firmly in place as I slapped her already flushed cheeks up to a glowing pink.

We have been friends ever since, and although distance ensures that we seldom meet it also means that the pleasure we take in each other is always fresh. I knew that Guy hadn't been the first to spank her, and that it had happened long before we met, but when I called her to ask for an interview she refused to provide more than teasing hints about what had happened. That left me with no choice but to visit her, and yet in any friendship that involves spanking there is always an easy way to make up for inconvenience. I arrived to find her out in her beautifully kept garden and wearing a loose summer dress, which she immediately lifted to show me that she was naked underneath. Half-an-hour later we began the interview, both thoroughly content, she now completely naked and sporting a distinctly pink bottom. Zoe –

"Right, you want me to tell you about my first spanking?"

"Yes, please."

"Okay. It was ages ago now. I was still in my teens, I think. Yes, I must have been, because that's when I knew Hairy Dave. He was one of the bikers who used to hang around at the Rising Sun, this pub on the corner of our street. I wasn't supposed to go there, so of course I did, and I wasn't supposed to talk to them, so of course I hung out with them whenever I could. They were up for that, and we used to drink with them and muck about together. I gave my first ever blow job to one of them, a guy called Pete, but you want to hear about the spanking, don't you?"

"A little extra colour won't hurt."

"It was just their attitude. Sex was just something you did, like drinking and riding fuck-off big motorbikes. I was flirting with Pete and I got him horny, so he took me round the back and pulled his cock out. He told me to suck it, but I didn't know what to do and refused, even though I wanted to, sort of, and I was sort of scared too. His cock was really big, and this dirty brown colour, with grease stains off his hands where he'd been working on his bike. He was half hard too, with this fat pink helmet just starting to stick out from his foreskin. I'd never seen anything so gross, or so horny. I was going to tell him to get lost, but then he said something I'll never forget – 'You got me like this, so fucking suck it.' That turned me on, in a weird way, like what he'd said meant I had to

93

do it, or maybe because I'd turned him on it was only right. I don't know, because I'd never heard about submissives or anything. I just knew I wanted to suck him. I had to suck him. So down I went, on my knees among these big silvery beer kegs, sucking on his big dirty cock, until he came in my face. It was really quick, maybe a minute, and it was like he was desperate to get there, wanking in my mouth with just the helmet between my lips, and telling me exactly how to do it. When he spunked it went all over my face as well as in my mouth. He laughed at me, because my face was all streaked with spunk, and then gave me this horrible oily rag that had been in his pocket and told me to clean up. I couldn't, of course, because I'd have been a bigger mess afterwards, so I nipped in the back of the pub and made a run for the Ladies, only I ran into the landlady in the passage and there's me with my face all streaked with spunk. She just looked at me and shook her head, that's all, I swear."

"I suppose she knew where her profits came from."

"That's for sure. They used to drink there all the time, and ride their bikes up and down the road. This was years ago, of course. It's a gastro pub now. So anyway, I thought, because I'd sucked Pete off, that there'd be something between us, but it didn't work that way. It made me one of their girls, but not his, and after that they were all really open with me, but dirty too, touching me up and everything. I didn't know if I loved it or hated it, but I kept coming back. That's what led to my spanking. I wanted to learn how to ride a bike, a motorbike. Most of them wouldn't let me touch their precious machines, but one of them, Hairy Dave, had an old wreck he liked to tinker with as well as his proper one. He said he'd

94

give me a go, but it was fucking huge, and you can imagine me on it, with my legs apart and my bum stuck out like I was riding a horse."

"Very pretty. What were you wearing?"

"Ripped up jeans, with quite a lot of bum showing, so yeah, I don't suppose I can blame him. He put his hand on my bum first, pretending to steady me, but really just out to grope my bum. They all knew it, and they were laughing, and then, when I fucked up on something, he gave me a smack. It was such a shock, not that it hurt, but he'd smacked my bottom, like I was a little girl or something, and it just went straight to my head, total outrage and a really, really desperate need for more. I told him to fuck off, but he just laughed and did it again, and again, and then he was spanking me in front of all his mates, with me mounted up on his motorbike with my bum sticking right out and half my cheeks showing through the rips in my jeans. He wasn't even holding me down, but I couldn't get off. I couldn't make myself stop it, and it just filled my head up right to the top. I started to cry, and he was laughing at me and calling me a cry baby, and still spanking me. I could have come, I really could, and you know I can when the spanking's just right, but he stopped, suddenly and went back to showing me how the controls worked. To him it was just a joke, no big deal, and that's what I came over when I did myself later, the way it was so important to me but just a laugh for him."

"That's very powerful, thank you."

Not Too Old for a Spanking – Jane Stewer

Anybody familiar with the West Country will immediately spot Jane as a Devon girl. She certainly looks the part of a

Devon girl, with beautiful thick hair, skin like the smoothest, richest cream and curves so opulent that I found great difficulty in not interviewing her cleavage. If I had difficulty keeping my eyes off her chest, then it was quite impossible to keep my hands off her bottom, treating her to a squeeze and a pat in the middle of a busy London street outside the pub where we'd had the interview. Considering what we'd been talking about for the previous hour I feel I was actually very restrained.

Usually, nowadays, she prefers to be the one dishing it out, preferably to a smartly suited businessman, while her ambition is to spank an MP, not as punishment, I hasten to add, but purely for fun. Nevertheless, for all her leaning towards the dominant role she's the sort of girl any red-blooded male would like to spank, or at least, any red-blooded, kinky male, and she has indeed been spanked, many a time.

My own first time with her is well worth relating. We'd organised a Victorian-style picnic, to be held in a secluded area of a well-known park which had better remain nameless. It was late July, the sun so hot that our elaborate costumes were soon unbearable, while the long grass hid us from all but the most determined of voyeurs. Clothes began to be unfastened, bodices opened and dresses discarded completely. Victorian underwear is cool and light, but covers far more than many a modern skirt and top combination, let alone a bikini, allowing the girls the pleasure of running around in their underwear without risking arrest. Victorian underwear is also designed to allow visits to the loo without having to disrobe completely, which means that the knickers allow easy access, either via a split at the back or a panel held up by buttons. Jane's were the sort that button, and, not to put too fine a point on it, they quite simply weren't up to the task of holding her in. One burst, a second burst, and before long she was bare bottom in the long grass. So I spanked her. What's a man to do?

Jane's own spanking story comes from the late 70s, a world away from modern attitudes, so much so in fact that as she told it I was reminded of Devon stories from during the Second World War rather than the county as it is now. She even used to be known as 'the maid', a West Country colloquialism for any girl or young woman that is now almost extinct. That was what they called her when she got her first job, as a clippy for the Devon General Bus Company, working a route along the south coast between Brixham and Paignton. She remembers it well, the smell of diesel in the depot, cider with her friends after work, the ill-fitting blue-grey uniform consisting of a jacket so short it left the lower part of her bottom showing in trousers that must have been designed for a man, in that while baggy and awkwardly long they were indecently tight across her cheeks. She also remembers Len, her driver, a big man in his sixties, close to retirement. Jane –

"He'd been on the buses since the 30s. It was his life. I can picture him now, sitting behind the wheel of his Routemaster, his massive body wedged into the driver's compartment, his bald head gleaming in the wet yellow light of the shed. He was a big man, and one of the most senior drivers, so everybody respected him, even the Inspectors."

"And how did he treat you?"

"Oh, nowadays he'd get sacked for inappropriate behaviour, for being a condescending, sexist pig, but back then that was normal, just the way an older, senior man would normally treat a young woman just starting out. But don't get me wrong. He wasn't nasty, that was just the way he was. If you'd told him it was wrong to call me the maid, or love, or to crack jokes with his mates about the way my trousers fitted, he wouldn't even have understood. He was a bit of an authoritarian too. He expected me to do as I was told, just because I was a lot younger than him."

"And a woman?"

"And a woman."

"Were you happy with all this?"

"Yes. I sometimes wish I'd stuck with it, but I was determined to get on in life. Now I have to spend my time worrying about deadlines and copy, and being polite to a load of Z-list celebrities who think they can write."

"But you have such a glamorous job. A lot of people would envy you."

"Bollocks. I hate the celebrity culture. I wish I'd stuck with being a clippy. It was such a simple life, and you know what, if I had I'd still have been doing it for less time than Len."

"You mentioned that he was close to retirement."

"Yes, and he hated it. His home life wasn't that good and he loved his work. He was somebody, the way he saw it, and once he'd retired there'd be nothing to do."

I learnt quite a lot over the next few minutes of our interview, about the Devon General Bus Company, about Len and his partially disabled wife, about Jane's hopes and fears as a young woman, but none of it strictly relevant. At length I managed to get back to the subject at hand.

"So how does this relate to your first spanking? Len did it, presumably?"

"Didn't he just, the dirty old bastard! No, that's not fair, not really, because I was really the one in control, not at first, maybe, but once the pretence that he was actually punishing me was gone, but let me explain."

"Sorry, carry on. So Len wanted to spank you and tried to pretend it was a punishment?"

"Yes, sort of. He always used to joke about it, saying that what I needed was a smacked bottom occasionally, that I wasn't too old for a spanking, that sort of thing. It was mainly when I was late, because I had to get up at some ridiculous hour and I've never been good in the mornings."

"Did you mind?"

"Yes and no. It used to embarrass me, especially when it was in front of the other drivers, which was most of the time, because he loved to show off to them, calling me 'his girl' and even telling the younger men off if they tried to chat me up. I know you're supposed to hate that sort of thing, and in a way I did, but it was flattering as well as embarrassing, because they made it very plain that as far as the crew went I was the sexy one. There are worse things."

"So he used to threaten to spank you?"

"Yes, but I knew he wouldn't actually do it, because he'd never have got away with it. This was the 1970s after all, not the 1870s!"

"But he did, in the end?"

"Yes! All the time I'd thought he was joking, just saying it to show off to his mates and keep me in my place, but the truth was he fancied me rotten. I didn't know this at the time, but for all his bravado he was really insecure underneath. He'd only ever had sex with his wife, I think, or at least since before the war, and none of that for years. He was desperate for me."

"So why didn't he proposition you?"

"Oh come on. He knew I'd turn him down, and I would have done. It didn't work like that."

"I can see that, so he decided to spank you because it was the only way he could get contact?"

"Something like that, but he was definitely into spanking. You should have heard the way he said the

99

word, as if he was smacking his lips over a prime rump steak."

"He was. No, never mind that. He can't have tricked you into accepting a spanking as a punishment, as you knew better, so?"

"I was late, again, but later than usual. I remember the day, some time in November. It was raining, and it was still dark when I arrived, but our Len had our bus halfway out of the shed, with an Inspector standing on the running board. I got told off, what nowadays would be called a formal verbal warning or some such bullshit. Len made a joke of it as we set off. I remember his exact words – 'Scared Mr Davy were going to have those tight trousers down were you, maid?'. I told him where to go, politely, and he answered – 'Any more of that, my girl, and I'll do it myself. You're not too old for a spanking'. That was his favourite phrase – 'You're not too old for a spanking'."

"So you used to answer him back?"

"Oh yes. There was always banter, but no question who was in charge. He didn't care who heard either; the other crew, passengers, anybody, except management, and they were hardly ever around."

"How did you feel about his threats to spank you? They must have made you think."

"This sounds outrageous nowadays, but it didn't really seem that big a deal, the idea of an older man spanking a younger woman to discipline her, that is. Sure, it was embarrassing and if I'd ever imagined it would really happen my time keeping would have been immaculate … or a lot better anyway, but I didn't see it as wrong. I suppose that's hard to understand?"

"Not really. It's just a different way of looking at

things. So he'd threatened to spank you in the morning, but that wasn't unusual and you had no idea he'd go through with it?"

"None. I don't suppose he would have either, only he got the perfect opportunity. The bus broke down, which they did quite often. It was on the Dartmouth Road, where it runs along behind the front, and we were stuck there for hours. In the end we got towed in, long after dark. I remember it like it was yesterday, the big empty shed with the buses lined up, two and three deep, how cold it was and the lights reflecting off the coloured puddles, with the smell of diesel in the air. I've never needed a tea so badly in my life. I made myself a mug and left Len to deal with Inspector Gurney. There was a sort of block of buses, and I went to the one in the very far corner, sipping my hot tea out of an old enamel mug and thinking about food."

"So the last thing on your mind was spanking?"

"Just about. I must have been daydreaming, because I remember I didn't notice Len until he put his weight on the footplate. It was gloomy, with just this very yellow light I'll always associate with that bus depot. He was sweating. I could see a bead of it on his forehead and I remember thinking that was odd because it was quite a cold evening. He was looking at me oddly too. I realise now that he was struggling with guilt and doubt, but at the time I just thought Gurney had been giving him gyp and he wanted to take it out on me in turn."

"You thought he was angry?"

"Yes, and believe me there was nothing guilty or doubtful about his voice when he spoke to me. 'Time for that spanking, my girl' – he said, and he wasn't joking. I could just have walked away. I could have

101

screamed for Inspector Gurney, only it wouldn't have done me any good, because he'd gone next door to talk to the mechanic, as Len knew perfectly well. Anyway, I could have left, but instead I tried to talk my way out of it, which was really as good as an admission that I was prepared to accept it."

"So he didn't manhandle you at all?"

"He didn't have to. I was trying to make excuses, and yes I was saying things like he didn't have the right, but I was badly flustered and I think he'd guessed he had me if he only kept his cool. We were in a Routemaster – some of the buses were older – and you probably remember that the seats nearest the entrance on the lower deck went along instead of across?"

"Yes. I can see where this is going. The perfect place to dish out a spanking!"

"Yes, and I'd sat on one side to drink my tea! He sat down on the other, on the edge of the seat so that his legs stuck out, making a lap. I stopped talking, just staring at his legs with my mouth open as I thought of what he was going to do to me, and he was. I'd given in, and I still don't know why. Maybe it was because he was so firm about it, as if I had no choice. He must have realised too, from the next thing he said – 'Come on, maid. The sooner you get in position the sooner it will be over'. So I went, across his knees for a spanking. I've never felt so small in my life, and you're not going to believe this, but I genuinely thought he was just going to discipline me. In fact I don't really know what I thought. I was completely confused, and then his arm had come around my waist and he'd begun to fiddle with the button of my trousers. I hadn't realised he meant bare, and I knew full well it would be my knickers as well as my trousers. It was a horrible shock, but I didn't try to get up. I told him not to, but he ignored me, and when I felt that button pop … I don't know, it just made me feel so weak. I was telling myself it was because he was in authority, that he had a right to spank me, but I knew it was a lie. Not that it made any difference what I thought, because he was tugging my uniform trousers down at the back and he'd caught my knickers too, so down they all came. I could just imagine how my bum would look, sticking up all round and bare in that dull yellow light. And he began to spank me, really firm swats right across my cheeks, and all the time telling me what a bad girl I was and how badly I needed what I was getting, and how he was just the man to do it, and how he should have done it a long time before, but most of all his favourite phrase – 'You're not too old for a spanking'. Now I realise that he was doing it because it turned him on, but at the time when I felt him start to go hard against my hip I thought it was just because he had my bare bum to spank and maybe because I was wriggling about a bit and rubbing on him. I knew he was going to want satisfying though, and I started to struggle. That only made him worse. The spanking got harder and I started to wriggle harder, until he was clinging onto me and I was thrashing about like a mad thing, with my legs going up and down and my fists thumping on the floor of the bus. I only made it worse for myself, going forward so that my bum was stuck right up in the air with my cheeks wide open so that he could see everything."

"That's quite a spanking."

"It was, believe me. It went on for a long time too. I don't know how long, but by the time he stopped my bum was so hot. I was dizzy from having my head upside down, and more confused than ever because I was incredibly turned on, in a way I never had been before. I still felt really resentful for what he'd done to me, but at the same time I wanted to please him. I was telling myself he was going to make me do it anyway so I might as well get it over with as I unzipped him, but that was a lie too. The truth was he'd meant to spank me and pretend it was a genuine punishment, so he was amazed when I took his cock out and put it in my mouth. So was I! I could hardly take in what I was doing, sucking on some dirty old man's cock when he'd just spanked me, but it felt so right. He was big too, and already hard, this great thick pole of flesh sticking up out of his bus driver's trousers. I'd pulled his balls out too, and I remember the hair tickling my chin as I tried to take him right in. He wouldn't fit, and it was making my jaw ache, but he soon got me by the hair, holding me in place on his cock and whispering to me about what a good little maid I was, telling me he was going to spank me regularly in the future, and how I wasn't to stop whatever happened. I didn't, and I swallowed for him."

"And did he spank you regularly in the future?"

"Yes, but it wasn't the same as that first time."

Knickerless – Celeste Brown

One popular theory used to explain the desire to be spanked, and for sexual submission in general, is that it's a way for people in stressful, decision-making positions to shed their cares once the day's work is done. Sometimes this is true, and certainly for Celeste Brown. In day to day life she is the very image of the modern businesswoman, brisk, efficient and quite used to taking decisions that affect the lives of hundreds of people. She looks the part too, with striking red hair cut short and neat, glasses, heels, a smart city suit and an air that suggests she has just stepped out of an important business meeting. New York and Frankfurt are as familiar to her as London, while she drives a 6-series BMW and thinks nothing of dining at restaurants where most of us would blanch at the cost of a bottle of water. She also likes to be spanked.

I found this out because she chooses to get the discreet discipline sessions she needs from one of my fellow old-school spankers, Stephen, and after a little gentle persuasion he got her to agree to meet me, and him, in a quiet gastro pub not far from her Surrey home. Had I not been used to women who prefer to keep their private tastes very firmly to themselves I would never have guessed that she was into spanking, but within a few minutes of our meeting she was happily explaining to me that the best way to thank a man for punishing her was by sucking him off, something many girls agree on and which she claims to be particularly good at. Sadly I was unable to test this claim, but she certainly provided a memorable first spanking story, and an unusual one in that she didn't start to fantasise about spanking until she was in her thirties. Celeste –

"I can't remember when I first began to feel the need to be spanked, but it crept up on me gradually, growing stronger and stronger. At first I tried to put my feelings aside, but I couldn't resist searching on the net. What I found fascinated me, and made me feel better about what I wanted, so I quickly realised I was going to have to do something about my desires. Not that it was easy, because I had to be very circumspect with work, but I couldn't resist and I knew that if I didn't go through with it I'd end up regretting my decision. I created an online persona, honest but anonymous, designed to allow me to meet somebody in the flesh without them really knowing anything about me. It's harder than you might think, but eventually I managed to find a man whose tastes seemed to be compatible with my own."

"Which are?"

"To be spanked. I hadn't really gone much further than that, but I did know I wanted a man who would take control of me. Charles, we'll call him, had that, although it was a bit like a job interview, or as if he was ticking off boxes to make sure I suited him. I thought that was just a pose at first, or the way he was online, but when I finally spoke to him on the phone it was the same. That was quite exciting, in a way, because it made me feel as if I was being treated like a puppet, but it was annoying too. Stephen is much better. He made me laugh and then made me suck his cock in the Gents toilets."

"But you still agreed to meet Charles?"

"He was the best of those I'd talked to online, but it's harder than you might think to find a good spanker."

"Not at all. Most women say the same. Where did you meet Charles?"

"At a hotel near Gatwick Airport. I was flying out to Frankfurt and he lived quite nearby, in Brighton, so it was the ideal opportunity. We arranged to meet in the lobby, and believe me it took a lot of courage even to approach him. I'd never even been on a blind date before, but he took control immediately and I fell in with it, well, after a fashion. He'd ordered me to wear a skirt and stockings, and I'd obeyed, but his first instruction, before he'd even bought me a drink, was to go into the loos, remove my knickers and bring them back to him. I went, feeling pretty embarrassed, because I hadn't really thought it out. For a start I was wearing pink ones with hearts all over them, very girly, but it wasn't until I'd got them off that I realised that the tag at the back said XL. They were from … I'd better not say, I suppose, but it's a design house who're used to fitting out catwalk models. I suppose I was just flustered, but I couldn't bear the thought of him thinking I had a big enough bum to need XL knickers, so I tried to get the label off. I didn't have any scissors or anything like that in my bag, so I had to use my teeth. It took ages, and by the time the horrible thing finally came off the back of my knickers were wet. You can imagine my embarrassment, but the last thing I wanted was for him to think I wouldn't do as I was told, so back I went and gave him my knickers. I must have been as red as a beetroot, and after all that he just scrumpled them up and put them in his pocket."

"I bet he'd have loved to know about your discomfort. I know I would."

"I hadn't really made that connection at the time, so I didn't tell him, not even afterwards, but it did get to me. I felt small and off-balance, and I was desperate for him simply to take control. He did, first asking me if there was a good desk in my room. When I asked why he wanted to know he told me that he was going to bend me over it and spank me. That got me very excited, and for all his cool I must have been getting to him as well, because he told me we were going up after just one drink. He made me follow him up, two paces behind him, and I was sure everybody we passed would know what was about to happen to me. I was shaking so badly I could barely get the key in the door, but he was perfectly cool about it all. The moment we were inside he took the best chair and told me to strip. I wasn't sure if he wanted me to just undress, or dance for him, or what, but he told me exactly what to do, which order to take off my clothes, and when I was nude to open a bottle of wine."

"Very controlling."

"Very controlling indeed. He made me serve it to him in the nude and on my knees, then drank some while I knelt on the floor at his feet, not even allowed to move. He lingered over his glass, watching me all the time, and when he'd finished he ordered me to undress him. I did as I was told, and by the end he had a huge erection, but when I went to lick him he slapped my face and said – 'I didn't tell you to do that. Get over the desk for your spanking'. I went, and he started to spank me, hard. It was exactly what I'd wanted, but I hadn't realised it would hurt so much."

"But you didn't try to get up?"

"No, I stayed down. I wanted to be right for him, and it was working. After about twenty smacks he felt my cunt, which was wet, and asked me if I was enjoying my spanking. I admitted I was and he gave me another twenty or so, then ordered me to kneel to him again, with my heels pressed into my smarting bottom. He let me have some wine – it was white, and very cold – then told me to suck his cock. That was really nice, but before he came he pulled out and did it in my face, then made me kneel back and put my hands on my head with his come dripping down my face and over my tits. He told me what a slut I looked."

"That's one advantage of starting with an experienced man. He obviously knew how to handle you. Was that the end, or did he let you come?"

"Not then. He wasn't finished with me. He made me kneel over a footstool with my bottom stuck right up in the air and started spanking me again. Then he pulled his belt out of his trousers and beat me. That really hurt. I was grateful when he stopped."

"But you still stayed down?"

"You keep asking that. Are you supposed to get up?"

"Not really, but it's an option. You're very obedient."

"This was my first time!"

"Charmingly naive them, but do go on. So he beat you hard?"

"Yes. I was grateful when it stopped and he made me stand up and put my hands on my head while he went to his case. He took out an inflatable dildo, a black one."

"How big?"

"Not scarily large, but it was inflatable and I was pretty sure I knew where it was going, because he'd only touched my cunt once but he seemed obsessed with my bottom. I was right too. He made me kneel on the bed and started stroking my cheeks very gently to make me relax, lubricated me and then inserted the dildo into my anus. He said that if I cried out or wriggled he'd take his belt to me again. Then he started to pump up the dildo. I managed to hold back, and when he did it the second time, but the third time I started to whimper. I just couldn't help it. He left the dildo in, started to beat me again and told me he wasn't going to stop until I'd come. I had no choice but to rub myself off in front of him, with the dildo still up my bottom, which was the most embarrassing thing I've ever done, but when I came it was like no other orgasm I've had before."

With her Husband Watching – Chrissie

I met Chrissie and her husband George at a dinner party

shortly after I had begun to write this book. All my close friends know what I like, otherwise they wouldn't be close friends, but I could sometimes wish they'd be a little more discreet in company. This was one of those occasions, at least initially, although looking back I can only look on what happened with a smile. The dinner was a black-tie affair hosted by an old college friend who is now a barrister. Most of the other guests were also in the legal profession, including George, a very serious, even stern, man who shared my friend's chambers. George was with his wife, a petite, exceptionally slender blonde in a clinging black dress that did rather more than hint at a perfect little cherry of a bottom. I found it hard to keep my eyes off her, especially as she proved to be not only charming but distinctly flirtatious. Our host, very much of the old school but with a wicked streak, came over to make formal introductions, remarked on George's hopes of becoming a QC and then quite casually stated that I was a writer currently working on a book about girls' first spankings. I nearly choked, but there was method in my friend's madness, as I'd barely begun my attempt to dab the champagne off my shirt front when George responded by telling me he spanked his wife and asking if I would like to include her first experience in my book. So here it is, not, I hasten to add, taken at the dinner party, but in private at a later date. Chrissie –

"George started to spank me as soon as we met, in 2006. He made it very plain from the start, that if I wanted to be with him I had to accept regular spankings. I like that in a man, honestly, so I let him. I had never been spanked before and it felt strange being taken down across his knee and having my dress pulled up and my knickers taken down, just as if it he was really going to punish me. Part of me wanted to resist, that's the social conditioning, but a much bigger part of me felt that it was completely natural. I really enjoyed the actual spanking too. He held me tight and wouldn't take any nonsense, but he was gentle at first so my bottom was warm before the smacks got hard."

"So it was a proper spanking?"

"A proper spanking!? Yes. With George it's always a proper spanking, and I love every minute spent across his knee. It's not just the excitement either. I feel a complete sense of relief when I am being spanked, and for a few hours afterwards, nursing a sore little bottom. I love having a glowing red bottom, and the feeling of well-being that it gives me. Only later did I discover that this was caused by something called 'endorphins' that the body produces to combat pain."

"That and in your case also the psychology of being punished by somebody you love, I suspect."

"Yes. Anyway, let me tell you about my first spanking from a stranger. George absolutely loves having me over his lap and giving me a good spanking, just as I love him spanking me, but after a while he decided he would like to see it from a distance, as it were. One day, to my surprise and horror, he said he wanted to take me somewhere, to another man, to watch me having my bottom spanked. I wasn't at all sure about it at first, but eventually I agreed. He organised it all, very carefully to make sure he got the right man for me. I felt more nervous every day, especially when he told me he'd found someone suitable on a naughty website. At first I couldn't believe it was really going to happen, but I should have known George better. He never backs out. I would have done, I think. I remember, in the taxi over to this man's apartment, feeling that I might jump out of the taxi and run away at any moment!"

"But you didn't, and I suspect you didn't really want

to?"

"No, but I did need George to make me feel secure. Still, even after we arrived and as I was getting changed into a naughty spanking outfit I could not believe what I was doing."

"Describe your outfit, please."

"George had chosen it for me. I had high, strappy heels, pink and white, white hold-ups, matching knickers and bra in pink and white, all very snug fitting, and a pink mini-skirt and halter top, all very different from what I usually wear. When I came out the man, let's call him Bob, said I looked sweet. I could see he was turned on, but he was calm as well, and he made the whole experience really delightful. First he gave me flowers and a kiss, just a peck. Then he sat down on his sofa and pulled me down ever so gently across his knee. I was shaking and I could barely believe what was happening to me as he turned up my skirt, and as for when he took down my knickers … It was nearly too much, and all the time with George watching and able to see everything as another man got me ready for a spanking punishment."

"I can imagine."

"He started to spank me, ever so gently. It was almost too gently! But he built it up the way skilled spankers do, to very hard smacks that had me wiggling my bottom and left me very red and sore. It felt wonderful, and he fully understood that it wasn't going to go any further, so in the end it was a really wonderful experience. That's what started it, and since then I've been spanked by literally dozens of men, always with my husband watching. For the most part it has been really enjoyable and George and I have met some very lovely and very interesting people. Only on a couple of occasions has there been an idiot who did not know how to spank or who was clearly just a nasty sadistic sod! But even that was not a problem because George simply stepped in and stopped everything."

"You make a great team, and you, Chrissie, are a spanker's dream, if I may say so."

We had agreed in advance that I would be allowed to join the privileged group of men who have spanked Chrissie in front of her husband, so with the interview done I took her across my knee. She looked wonderfully demure in a cream-coloured roll-neck sweater and white slacks that clung to the shape of her bottom, not overtly sexual but enticing to say the least. I took my time, spanking her on the seat of her slacks and treating myself to a squeeze of her firm little bottom before getting her bare. She was very obliging, lifting her tummy to allow me to unfasten her slacks and pull them down to expose lacy white panties that seemed to have been painted on to her perfect cheeks. I knew I was allowed to pull them down, in fact it was expected of me, but again I felt no need to rush and spent a while enjoying her bottom, stroking as much as spanking. My smacks were getting firmer and she had begun to react, her skin beginning to grow pink and the occasional soft sigh escaping her lips. All the while George was watching, benevolent, amused and clearly well pleased with the sight of his wife being spanked across another man's knee. His expression barely flickered when I told her I was going to take her panties down, and once again she obliged by lifting her hips to make it easier for me to strip her.

With Chrissie's bottom bare and the pretty white panties inverted around her thighs I went back to spanking, now with her rosy cheeks pushed up and parted, her sighs growing deeper and her feet beginning to kick a little in response to the smacks. I could have gone on for hours, and

113

so, it seemed, could she, but George finally glanced at his watch and pointed out that she'd been over my knee for more than half-an-hour. Chrissie got up, rubbing her bottom but in no hurry to pull her knickers back up. Her face was wreathed in smiles and she gave a long, happy sigh before she spoke. Chrissie –

"That was just what I needed. Now I'm going to be happy all day. Do you know, I just feel sorry for all the women who resist letting men spank them. They don't know what they're missing!"

Whipped in the Woods – Rachel Jeffries

I met Rachel through a fellow spanking enthusiast. They are regular playmates and both as thoroughly dedicated to the art as anybody I've ever met. She knew who I was, and my reputation, so that we'd barely been introduced before she'd begun to speak to me with the same playful, purposeful insolence she uses on her boyfriend. That could only mean one thing, she was angling for a spanking, and despite being in similar situations a hundred times before that still makes my pulse race. Unfortunately we were in a busy West End bar at the time, and while spankings have been dished out in pubs I prefer not to risk a night in the cells for the sake of applying discipline on the spot. That could wait, but I did arrange an interview.

Rachel is soft, blonde and full of fun, also completely at ease with what she likes to do, all of which promised well. I went to see her at the smart London townhouse she shares with a large brown cat and was quickly installed in the most comfortable seat, my notebook in hand as we swapped spanking stories. She had so many that it was a little difficult to get her to focus on the first, but we got there eventually. Rachel –

"You need to know the back story first, because I'd known John for twelve years before he spanked me."

"I'm surprised. I'd imagined you as an early starter."

"Oh, spanking had always fascinated me, but I can't bear to have to ask for it and a lot of men won't do it even if you do."

"That amazes me. I'd have thought it was just good manners to give a lady what she wants?"

"So would I, but a lot of men don't see it that way. My husband certainly didn't."

"So you were married?"

"Yes, but Phil wasn't into spanking. He couldn't cope with it at all, but let's come back to that. I was telling you about John. I'd been studying in Italy and had come back to work in England. He was a colleague. I was used to sunbathing without very much on, and I like to run around naked as much as possible, so I think he picked up on the way I dressed. He used to give me a lift to the station after work, so at the end of the day I'd go up to his office. We used to joke with each other, teasing, and one time he had a staple gun and stapled my dress to his desk."

"He stapled your dress to his office desk? Why?"

"Because it was really low cut and it made the front pull down so he could see I didn't have a bra on. I didn't have any knickers on either, as he found out when he pulled up the back of my dress. It was a dominant gesture too, I can see that now, and he could have spanked me. I wish he had, but he didn't, not then. He just started to talk, telling me how he and his wife Rose were into naturism and group sex. We got into it, Phil and me and he and Rose, and often had foursomes at their house. He liked to dominate Rose, and to embarrass her, telling us how he'd spanked her and how pink her bum had been afterwards, but that was as far as it went. In the end they moved to Australia, which would have been the end of it, only when his parents died he had to come back several times to sort out the estate. He used to stay with us, and one night he told us how they'd met another swinging couple in Australia and that Rose had caned him in front of them at a dinner party. Phil couldn't deal with that at all, so what I'm sure John had meant to be a really high moment ended up in embarrassed silence. It was a really hot day and we were eating outside, so I cleared the table and went indoors. John followed me and in the kitchen his eyes lit on my container of wooden spoons. I'd gone to the sink, and he came up behind me and whispered into my ear, telling me how he'd like to spank me and how much he'd enjoy using the biggest spoon on my bottom."

"Were you surprised, or shocked?"

"No. It was something I'd thought about a lot, and I'd already guessed the evening was going to end in sex. Sure enough, later on Phil suggested I might like to take John upstairs, but as soon as we were in the bedroom he told me to go back down and fetch the wooden spoon. I was shaking really badly, and thinking to myself – 'This is for real!'. I was feeling cheeky, but I was a little bit scared too, so I brought him back the smallest spoon. He sent me straight back down, telling me to get the proper spoon, the one he meant. I knew which it was, the biggest, the one he'd already threatened me with. I've still got that spoon."

At this point Rachel broke off to go into the kitchen. She came back with a wooden spoon, perfectly ordinary except that it was worn to a stump. I assumed she was joking, although she is such a tease that it's hard to tell. Throughout the interview she had been dropping hints and passing cheeky remarks, which made it extremely difficult to keep up. She also talks so fast that my fingers were sore and I was very glad of the break, which allowed me to wiggle some circulation back into them. After another coffee we settled back down to the interview. Rachel –

"I thought he was going to spank me, over the knee, which is the way I'd always imagined it. I was a bit worried that Phil would hear, but John told me to strip, which was easy as all I had on was a light dressing gown, then to lie on the floor, on my back with my legs apart. I wasn't sure what he was doing, but I did as I was told. He smacked me between my legs, right on my clit. That really hurt, and it wasn't what I wanted at all, but then he passed me the spoon and made me ask for a spanking. Now I was sure I was going to get it, but instead of bending me over he made me stand up and started to smack my breasts. I was so frustrated, but after he'd made love to me he promised that I'd get a proper spanking the next day if I could arrange to be alone."

"So he knew he wasn't giving you what you wanted?"

"Oh yes, he knew, and to be fair it was because Phil might have heard."

"So Phil was perfectly happy for John to have full sex with you but not for him to spank you?"

"Yes. Phil never could handle spanking. In the end, when I asked for it, he told me I was a pervert. I have never had sex with him again. But getting back to John, we'd arranged to drive out to the country together the next day and Phil agreed. Breakfast seemed to take for ever, and the drive out into the

117

country, but we soon found a mini car park with nobody about. We began to walk, across fields and over stiles, until John decided to sit down on one and put me across his knee. I'll never forget how it felt, to go down like that, so very vulnerable as my dress was lifted and my bottom exposed for all the world to see. He didn't start to spank immediately, but gave me a gentle rub, which only made my feelings stronger before the sudden burst of hard smacks. I tried hard not to wriggle or cry out, but just as I was about to give in to the pain we heard voices and had to stop. We walked on again, now with my bottom hot under my dress and urgent for more. So was he. He made me go in among the bushes and touch my toes, turned my dress up again and I was introduced to the leather belt, only to get disturbed again before he'd given me more than a dozen smacks. I was feeling desperately frustrated, but we were about to start again when we realised the people who'd been following us were still about, so I suggested we climb the fence into a private wood. How's that for sealing my own fate?"

"Fairly typical, I'd say."

"I needed it, and I got it. We went right in, despite the brambles, until we found a glade with a silver birch growing to one side. I was made to strip naked and put my hands against the tree with my feet braced apart and my bottom stuck right out. He took off his belt again and began to beat me, really hard, a proper thrashing. I was so high I hardly felt it, not as pain. He even turned me around and whipped my breasts, leaving thick, red welts all over my skin. I think he wanted to make me cry, but I was too high for that, even when he'd beaten me black and blue. It took my bruises two weeks to go down."

"That must have hurt if he had you?"

"There was no sex, not ordinary sex, not that time, and a couple of days later he went back to Australia. That wasn't the only session though. He took me to the Janus shop and bought a cane, which he used on me at his son's flat. It was very hard, so hard I still have mixed feelings about it, and I've never really liked the cane since. Once he'd gone I thought it would all be over, but he made me talk to Rose on the phone and describe what he'd done to me. He also advised me to put an ad into one of the CP contact magazines, and that led on to plenty more encounters, as you know. Oh, and I'd typed it all out for you in advance, so you needn't have bothered taking all those notes."

She had, but although my fingers were aching badly from my frantic scribbling I still managed to put her across my knee and deliver the bare-bottom spanking she quite clearly wanted, and deserved.

Gentle but Firm – Emily Evans

I came across Emily quite by chance. She had heard that I was writing this book from an open-minded but not especially kinky friend. He put us in touch and I gladly accepted the opportunity to interview her, more gladly still as he described her as blonde and beautiful. That was no exaggeration, as I discovered when I visited her South London flat, while she was as uninhibited as she was beautiful, even giving me a brief twirl to show how snugly her tight blue jeans fitted her neatly rounded little bottom. We talked for a while, I explaining the book and she telling me how her boyfriend had introduced her to the swinging scene but that she never played unless he was there. As he wasn't, this was clearly a hint that this would not be one of those interviews which ended up with the subject over my knee, which was a shame but when it comes to spankings I'm a great believer in waiting patiently until the time is right. She also explained to me that she saw spanking as foreplay, a naughty thrill to spice up her sex life rather than something to do for its own sake, and also as something sensual. The idea of being punished didn't appeal, while she didn't even view accepting a spanking from a man as a submissive act. Emily –

"I know that's why some people like it, but for me it's all about the feeling. But I was going to tell you about my first time, and still the best. Me and Dave were at a sex club where two TVs were putting on a show, one spanking the other. The one doing the spanking obviously knew what he – or she, I suppose – was doing, and he was getting an amazing reaction. His – or her ..."

"Go for "her". She'd probably prefer that."

"Okay. Her friend was over a whipping stool with this little tarty dress she had on turned up to show a pair of see-through nylon panties. His cock – her cock I suppose – looked as if it was about to burst out it was so hard, and she was moaning and gasping as if she was about to come. I started to wonder if I'd feel the same. The TV doing the whipping was really patient, and kept bending down to whisper in her friend's ear. She was using her hand, mostly, but also a whip, a flogger made of suede, and not just spanking but stroking and tickling. In the end the girl being whipped came in her pants, and by then I knew I had to try it."

"But it wasn't something you'd thought about before?"

"No. I'd never made a connection between spanking and sex at all, but it looked amazing, and just watching had got me really horny. Dave was keen too, so he let me ask the TV, Joanna …"

"Hang on. Joanna, quite tall, honey blonde hair, usually in a skirt so short she might as well not bother?"

"That sounds like her. Do you know her?"

"I know of her. She seems to have spanked her way through half the girls in the country, and quite often for their first times."

"She's very good. I asked if she'd spank me and she made sure I really wanted it first, but once she was sure it was okay she was firm with me. Gentle but firm. She was gentle with the spanking too, making me bend over the whipping stool so I had no choice but to stick my bum right out, but then asking both me and Dave if it was all right to lift my dress. All I had on underneath was a thong, and she left that up and started to spank me, ever so gently. It was too gently if anything, but a lovely feeling, warm and tingly, which made me want to stick my bum up for more. I got it, gradually harder, for ages, until I was glowing behind and really turned on. She used the flogger too, and after maybe twenty minutes – a long time anyway – she asked if I'd like to be caned. I was a little scared, but I let her and she gave me two strokes. They stung, but I was so turned on it really felt quite nice, so I asked for two more, then another two, which left my bottom so hot and gave me the most amazing feeling. I hadn't come, but I wanted to, so when Joanna offered me a massage I just quickly checked with Dave and then accepted. She was really good at that too. First she had me strip, naked, then lie down on a massage table in another room. Just like the spanking she took it really slowly, stroking my neck and back, and asking first if she could part my legs and then if she could touch my cunt. I wanted it far too badly to say no and Dave loves to see me get like that for somebody else, so I let it happen. Joanna was using these amazing finger sheaths made of delicate wires, so it was like being tickled and scratched at the same time, very subtle and very slow, so it took ages, but when I did come it was truly spectacular, one of the best orgasms I've ever had. That was my first spanking, so you see why I like it?"

"Yes, absolutely, and I can see that I'm going to have to track down this Joanna."

Spanking the Stars – spanking accounts from the girls we all know and love

THE WORLD OF ENGLISH spanking is an institution, with imagery and ideas that go back many, many years and derive from the collective experiences of many, many people. That imagery and those ideas are too firmly established to be easily influenced. New ideas are rare and seldom if ever carry the impact of the classics, and so it is that the stars of the spanking scene are those who best reflect it and best express those classic scenarios. Many names come to mind, too many to be easily listed. Among the men involved, George Harrison Marks of *Kane* magazine certainly stands out, and perhaps Ivor Gold of Red Stripe, but it is the girls we remember. Over the years many hundreds of women must have graced the pages of magazines and the screens of our TVs and computers with their bare, red bottoms and their enticing expressions. The vast majority of them were and are genuine spankings enthusiasts, paid or otherwise. There has never been a shortage of willing volunteers.

I have never been deeply involved with the commercial side of spanking – despite appearing on the cover of *Kane* Issue 101 with the delectable Leia-Ann Woods – but I have been privileged to know many of those who were and are. Among these I have encountered a handful of men and a very few women who were simply there to exploit the situation, but nearly all have not only been genuine enthusiasts but a pleasure to know. Choosing who to include

123

was not easy, but some names do stand out.

No book on spanking would be complete without a mention of Bettie Page, the most famous 50s pin-up girl of all, bondage bunny and iconic spanking model. There is no doubt that her beauty and her playful but often contradictory style have exerted a strong influence on popular culture and eroticism in the West, perhaps more so even than Marilyn Monroe. At once naughty and nice, sweet and fiery, coy and daring, she filled the world with delightful, sexy images that are popular today, sixty years later. From what is known we can only be sure that her own sexuality and her attitude to sex in general changed across her lifetime, as it usually does, but it seems fair to say that she thoroughly enjoyed modelling, including being spanked. I have no idea when her first time would have been, but her first recorded spanking was probably in 1952, when she began to work for Irving Klaw, another major name in the development of fetish imagery.

There were plenty of spanking models before Bettie and yet more after, but no name has stuck in the public imagination in the same way, and it must be that there are many hundreds, if not thousands, of women who owe their enjoyment of a well smacked bottom to Bettie Page. No other model has been as influential, but one does come close: Lynn Paula Russell, better know as Paula Meadows. If there is one woman who can be said to represent the spirit of English spanking it is Paula. Model, writer and artist, she lived and breathed spanking erotica for more than twenty years until her recent retirement. She has been the subject of many a photo set and written a considerable amount, mainly as editor of *Februs* magazine, but I suspect that she will be mainly remembered for her artwork. Technically brilliant, she always seemed to capture the very essence of a spanking situation, not only the erotic, but comedy, shame, apprehension and all the other emotions that come together to create a classic spanking scenario. Whatever situation she chose to depict, she always had an extraordinary ability to key in directly to my fantasies, as if she and I had discussed the piece before she set to work. What that reflects is the established imagery of English spanking, which all enthusiasts share, but nobody was better at bringing it out that Paula.

My first memory of Paula comes from an issue of *Janus* magazine. I was immediately captivated, not only by her petite beauty and exquisitely feminine bottom, but because of the way the piece shows her interacting with what is being done to her. I'd seen spanking magazines before, with any number of girls being punished, but the over-riding impression was either of spanked wives and girlfriends doing it for fun or paid models. Paula combined the two, and in many ways opened my eyes to the full possibilities of the world of spanking.

Sadly she declined an interview, having moved on from the world of spanking. However, her story has been published more than once, including her first spanking at the hands of an experienced French enthusiast.

For more than ten years Paula was undoubtedly the best known British spanking model, but every star is eclipsed in time, and in this case by a girl who for many spanking enthusiasts still represents perfection.

The Perfect Blonde – Lucy Bailey

You don't see so much of Lucy Bailey nowadays, when everything is focussed on the internet, but in the high days of video she was quite simply *the* spanking queen. With her pert, blonde good looks and mischievous attitude she had every man who liked to redden up a girl's bottom at least half in love with her, and not a few of the women. I don't blame them.

It's hard to define exactly what made her stand out from the crowd. She's small, blonde and bouncy, with a divine

125

bottom, firm but ever so slightly fleshy on her tiny frame, a spanker's dream. She has just the right character, a blend of innocence and cheek, playful but with a touch of reserve, sexy with more than a touch of impudence. She always seemed to be in need of a spanking. Yet for all that I suspect that what made her special was that when you saw Lucy on video, and when you met her, you got the impression that if the circumstances were right you might get to spank her too.

My first memory of her is very clear indeed, because she was to all intents and purposes stark naked. I'd gone to collect Penny from a girls-only party but turned up far too early and found myself sitting in the car and twiddling my thumbs for over an hour. Normally I'd simply have been bored, but this was agonising. There were a dozen or so kinky girls in a flat just a few yards away. My imagination was running wild and knowing that Penny would give me all the juicy details later that evening only made it worse. She knew I was there as well, but showed no inclination to hurry up, so I was also thinking about the spanking she was going to get when we finally got home.

Eventually the door opened and a girl came out, not Penny but a small, pretty blonde in a long coat and black ankle boots. She glanced up and down the road, then at my car, ran over, said, "You must be Pete," and opened her coat. Underneath she was stark naked, and I had just an instant to take in a pair of little round tits topped by perky nipples, a taut belly and the V of her pussy between neatly turned thighs before she'd covered herself up and begun to walk away, only to swish aside her coat and flash her naked bottom. She was laughing as she ran off, and I was left with the image of that gorgeous, full-frontal flash and her lovely bare bum swimming before my eyes, which more than made up for that long, tedious wait. Penny had arranged it, but she still got spanked.

I didn't even know her name at the time, but soon found out as I had to endure over a month of Penny boasting about the fifteen girls she'd met at the party, Lucy included. They got on well and became regular playmates at both clubs and private parties, including one especially fine incident with both dressed as schoolgirls when Penny caned Lucy in front of their "class" and several hundred onlookers at a benefit for the Spanner Men. I didn't know her quite as well, and looking back over our records I discover that I was spanked by her and side-by-side with her before I got to deal with her myself.

That came nearly a year after we first met, at one of our own parties. She was in school uniform again, a favourite look for her and one that set her off to perfection, with tight white panties just peeping out from beneath a pleated tartan miniskirt. It was a busy party, and I forget what led up to the spanking, but I do remember picking her up under one arm to lift her clear of the ground, pulling down her panties to get her bare in front of the rest of our guests and spanking her until she apologised for whatever it was she had done. I also remember that she finished the evening stark naked after having her pussy shaved by another girl and her boyfriend.

At the time I was struck by her extraordinary confidence, especially for one so young, and the story of her first spanking reflects that. This was only a few months before we first met, and back in the early 90s things were very different. Lucy –

"I was always interested in being submissive from a very young age and was drawn towards spanking and bondage. Unlike men I'd never seen a porn magazine and there was no world-wide web back then so I had no idea that anyone else shared my desires. My fantasies all stemmed from romantic fiction stories like *Wuthering Heights* and *The Arabian Nights*, only in my versions the heroines always ended up getting a spanking. At the age of about nineteen I saw an add in *Loot* magazine to join a Spanking Club. It was called The Moonglow Club. So I rang up and went to an interview with a gentleman named George."

"You say that so casually. Most of the women I've interviewed wouldn't have dared, especially not at nineteen."

"I wanted a spanking."

"Fair enough. So you joined The Moonglow Club? I remember the Moonglow videos you did, especially the one in a cricket club. I think you were wearing a maid's uniform, but I do remember he spent ages spanking you on the seat of your panties before pulling them down. That was the best stripping I'd seen at the time, so he obviously knew what he was doing."

"He did, believe me, but I didn't. The interview was mainly to make sure I wasn't from the press, I think, and he didn't spank me, although I'd half been hoping he would, but I was invited along to their next event. It was at a house in South London. I turned up and was ushered into a room with three other girls. We sat waiting and talking, and that was the first time I'd spoken to other girls who liked to be spanked, and had been. You can imagine how I felt!"

"Knowing you, keen."

"Yes, I suppose so, but I was nervous too. That was mainly because we were called in one by one and I was last. I watched each girl go out through that door. I heard the talking and the men laughing, then the smacks and her cries as she had her bottom smacked. Then she'd come out looking flushed and show us her red bum. I was just about wetting myself when my turn came, but it was as if I was on automatic."

"What were you wearing, school uniform?"

"Yes, only not the one you like with the little tartan

skirt and white panties. George had said I'd make a good schoolgirl, but I didn't have much money and I didn't even know where to go to buy a sexy schoolgirl outfit. So I turned up in what I'd been wearing the year before in sixth form."

"The real thing?"

"Yes, and I know you'd like the details. A white blouse with my tie half undone like a St Trinian's girl, a knee-length pleated skirt, black shoes, white socks and big, bottle-green panties."

"I bet that went down well."

"It did. When I walked in I swear some of the men actually looked guilty. Shifty anyway, but like I said I was on automatic. I can't even remember which man did it, just the way he stuck his knees out to make a lap and patted his leg. Down I went, OTK for the first time in my life, and everything seemed to be in slow motion as he turned my school skirt up and began to spank me through my panties. It hurt, but I was in heaven. I could feel every smack and the way my bum was growing warmer, something I'd dreamt about so often but never experienced. It was the same with having my panties pulled down. I'd imagined the moment so many times, but actually to have a man do it to me was mind -blowing, just to feel myself going bare and to know I was showing everything to all those men, but I don't remember who they were, not one of them. Not that it matters. What mattered was the spanking, my first."

"But not your last."

"Not by a long way, not even that night. After our initial spankings me and the other girls were brought out individually and together to play out little scenarios and get punished both by the men and by each other, so my second ever spanking was from another girl. That went on for ages, and my bum got so hot that every time I was sent back to the waiting room I'd pull down my panties and stand with my cheeks pressed against the cold metal of an iron filing cabinet to try and cool them down. There was also a part where we were handed around the audience to be spanked over the knee by each person, and the event ended with us all lined up and severely caned."

"And you took it all, because you wanted it, or because you were being paid and you felt you had to?"

"Because I wanted it, but that's the funny part. I know this sounds really naive, but I didn't realise I was being paid. After the party was over George gave me an envelope with money in it, which was the last thing I was expecting, because I didn't just not realise that I was being paid for my services. I thought I'd have to pay him!"

"I'd have charged you."

"I bet you wouldn't, but I wouldn't have minded. It was so exhilarating, especially having a red hot bottom on the way home, and I was dripping down my legs with sexual excitement. I remember even the motion of the car on the way back was almost bringing me to orgasm and I knew I had to come or I was most likely going to crash. It was about three o'clock in the morning, so I turned into a side road and stopped. It was just some suburban street, but that made it even better as I turned my panties down and sat my hot bottom on the seat so I could remember how it had felt to be bare while I was spanked. I played with myself until I'd come at least three times and had to drive all the way back sitting in a wet patch. There was lots more masturbation for some time afterwards, because every time I thought of what had happened I wanted to come. So that was my first spanking and it's totally true."

"From you, I don't doubt it for a moment, but I think you have another important first."

"I do?"

"Yes. Do you remember the pony-girl club piece we did for Eurotrash?"

"When I stuck the tail up my bum? Yes."

"That's the one, but I gave you a warm-up spanking first, didn't I?"

"Yes. You were in your red hunting coat and that ridiculous wig that looked as if you'd got a guinea pig sitting on your head."

"Never mind the wig. That was a mistake. I spanked you, and the crew filmed it and showed you getting your spanking. You were in a PVC miniskirt and hold-up stockings, no knickers."

"If you say so."

"I have a photograph to prove it, taken from the rudest possible angle. The film crew didn't get such a rude view, but they did film you getting your spanking and they did show it. That was May of 1995, and it was shown a few weeks later, so unless I'm very much mistaken that means that you were the first girl ever to be spanked for pleasure on British TV, as opposed to an actress getting it. In fact I think it was a double first, because you stuck the plug of the tail up your bum and I think that was the first real anal penetration shown on British TV. You're a star."

I'm not one hundred per cent certain that the spanking I gave Lucy on Eurotrash was the first ever play spanking shown on British TV, but I can't think of an earlier one, although obviously there were plenty in films. I'd be interested to know if anybody remembers an earlier example.

The Perfect Brunette – Leia-Ann Woods

I don't suppose there are many spanking enthusiasts who haven't heard of Leia-Ann Woods, unless they don't have the internet or read the papers. She was involved in 2008's most notorious sex scandal, very definitely on the side of the angels, and it's probably fair to say that in all of Britain, if not the world, she is currently the woman most famous for enjoying having her bottom smacked. She is also beautiful, which no doubt added to her notoriety, elegant, willowy and delicate, but above all, poised, the result of years of ballet training. Her expression is cool and serene, occasionally mischievous but more often with a touch of quite unintentional hauteur, a look perhaps more suited to sexual dominance than submission, but one that makes her an absolute joy to spank.

Usually when I spank a girl my pleasure is more or less evenly divided between the physical – the sight of her body, her scent, touching her flesh and feeling her wriggle – and the mental – enjoying her reactions to what is being done to her; anticipation, apprehension, arousal and perhaps best of all, her embarrassment. For my first time with Leia, for all that she was barely twenty and gorgeous by even the most exacting standards, the mental aspect definitely had the edge. It was at The Night of the Cane, a club specialising in corporal punishment, the highlight of which was the annual caning competition. Leia-Ann was entered in the competition, which I was judging. I always prefer to test the mettle of entrants before the competition, and so suggested to her partner that she might benefit from a spanking. He agreed, and over my knee she went, at first clothed and then with her mini-dress lifted and her silky black knickers pulled down. Just to have her over my knee was a joy, and she was also perfectly obedient, but the real delight was in her open embarrassment and resentment for what was happening to her, so strong and so well expressed in her eyes that I ended up not only highly aroused but touched with guilt, not something that normally bothers me at all. Fortunately that guilt was short-lived, as I quickly discovered that she possesses an almost unrivalled enthusiasm for being spanked, or rather for both the prospect of being spanked and the after-effects. She hates the actual spanking, which makes her a sadist's dream, as we'll see. I wasn't the first, because she was a quick starter, although to judge by the opening of her interview not quite as quick as she might have liked. Leia-Ann –

"I wasn't spanked until I was nineteen."

"Anybody I know?"

"No. My first proper boyfriend, well, sort of boyfriend, because I was more into girlies at the time."

"Juicy details, please?"

"Nothing too juicy, I'm afraid, although when we were performing Swan Lake another girl and I always used to kiss before we went on. We used to pretend it was for luck, but really we were getting off on it, or at least I was! Then the director caught us. He was furious, not because we were kissing so much, but because I was kissing her and not him."

"We're not talking sisterly pecks on the cheek here, are we?"

"No, we're not. That's as far as it went though."

"What a pity. I'd love to see you get spanked in your ballet dress, or perhaps the pair of you, side by side with your bottoms bare and your colleagues watching as the director dealt with you. Okay, never mind that … You preferred girls. So were you a virgin?"

"No. I tried normal sex, with a man, because I was

worried that my sexual orientations and preferences were odd. But what I found odd was straight sex itself."

"But you had a boyfriend?"

"A sort of boyfriend. We'd been seeing each other for a while. I'd just finished my ballet and I'd gone home to Brighton to complete my A levels. He was in one of my classes. We went out, nothing serious. One night we were in this pub and I was in one of my particularly irritating moods, giving him a steady stream of quips and abuse. I think I must have been giving off some kind of kinky signal, but eventually he caught me up under my bum and lifted me over his shoulder in a fireman's lift, a wise move, as I could easily have run away and would have done if I'd known what he was up to."

"Which was?"

"He started to spank me, in front of everybody!"

"What were you wearing?"

"My typical outfit of jeans and skinny top, so not bare or anything, but he had my bum stuck right up in the air, so it was still seriously embarrassing, especially as a lot of the guys were egging him on."

"So your audience approved?"

"They seemed to. The men loved it, but it was harder to read the women. You never know with women if it's shock or delight."

"That's true. They say men have trouble expressing their emotions, but in edgy, erotic situations women are usually far harder to read. So he's got you over his shoulder and he's spanking you in the middle of a Brighton pub. What happened next?"

"He stopped and asked me if I was going to stop being a pain in the arse. I refused to answer, because I was completely mortified by the whole situation. I knew I was a pain in the arse, but he was showing off, trying to get me to admit it in front of everyone while I was spanked. The public humiliation was too much."

"So you didn't get any pleasure out of it at the time?"

"Not really. I'd fantasised about it so often, but not like that!"

"Yet the situation was almost classic?"

"Yes, and now my biggest fantasy is public humiliation. It obviously stems from that."

"And before that you'd seen it differently?"

"Yes. I was more general in my fantasies, and I still don't insist on one special thing. I'm glad of that, because it means that whatever I get it's not a disappointment. Some girls need it to be exactly right."

"And the spanking got to you eventually?"

"Oh yes. I don't enjoy being spanked, not the sensation of it. I know a lot of girls do, but I don't get that at all. It hurts! What I enjoy is the thought of it before and thinking about it afterwards."

Leia-Ann's attitude is by no means uncommon, and to me it makes perfect sense. After all, being spanked does hurt, at least at first, and for all the powerful psychological needs that surround it there's no escaping that pain. The public perception is very different, that those who like to be spanked desire the pain for its own sake, which is in fact much rarer. For others the pain is a barrier to be crossed before their endorphins kick in, but even then it's not so much that they're enjoying the pain as that the pain has turned to pleasure.

I rather enjoyed Leia-Ann's first experience, which conjured up a wonderful picture of her struggling helpless over her friend's shoulder with the denim-clad bottom the highest part of her body, and yet it was a great shame she hadn't been bare, or at very least had her jeans pulled down. There had to have been a first time for that as well, so I continued –

"Can you remember the first time you were spanked on the bare?"

"Yes, by Steve. We'd just started going out and we'd been to see the *Secretary*, you know, the film where Maggie Gyllenhall gets spanked."

"He spanked you in the cinema!?"

"No. It was in a public place, but not in public. Nobody got to watch."

"That's a shame. So what happened?"

"He'd told me not to talk during the film. I thought I'd done quite well. He didn't. After the film he waited until everybody had left and took me to the Gent's toilets. You can imagine my embarrassment, especially when he made me bend over the sinks and pulled my dress up. Somebody might have come in at any moment."

"Hang on, we need details. You said you were bare, so did he pull your knickers down or make you do it?"

"I didn't have any on. That was a rule. No knickers. It made for easy access."

"I see. So he made you wait like that, bent over the sink in a public loo with your bare bottom stuck out?"

"Yes, while he took his belt off. That was really erotic, just watching him and knowing it was for me. He gave me sixteen, real stingers."

"So more of a beating than a spanking?"

"Oh yes. He doesn't mess around."

136

Express Punishment – Nina Birch

Nina, no relation, is best known as Lady Nina Birch, one of Britain's most highly skilled and exacting Mistresses, with a very English style and a reputation for old-fashioned, no-nonsense female domination. She certainly looks the part, sexy yet stern, with her fine, womanly figure and an expression that suggests you're likely to be put across her knee for the slightest infraction. It would take a brave man to suggest that she ought to be the one to get her bare bottom smacked instead of his own, but the truth is that she enjoys being on the receiving end just as much as she enjoys dishing it out. Nevertheless, it felt slightly peculiar to be interviewing her about her first spankings in a room furnished as an old-fashioned study, with Nina sitting behind the desk and a school cane on the wall behind her, rather as if I were some particularly villainous boy who'd managed to turn the tables on his headmistress. That makes it all the more delicious when she freely admits to getting spanked. Nina –

"Oh yes, being spanked has been quite the norm for me, although I'll only allow a few select people to do it. You'd better put that in, or I'll be inundated by demands from dominant men."

"Of course, and it's nice to think that I'm one of the few. So it's not so much that you don't get spanked very often as that you're fussy about who does the spanking?"

"Yes, and I like it my way. Over the knee is my favourite position, for hand spanking, preferably with a mirror behind me, because I love the way my bottom turns red, and the burning hot feeling all over. It turns me on to touch my smacked flesh, and to see myself in the mirror with a red spanked bottom.

Really I prefer implements though. My first birching experience was from Lucy Bailey and it's still my favourite implement – hence the name."

"That's unusual. Not that many people have tried the birch, and a lot of those who have find it too severe."

"That all depends how it's done. Lucy made it feel really sensual, and I had a businessman friend I used to see who always bought fresh birches with him ranging between six and fifteen stems. He would start very lightly birching me and would birch me solidly for ages, gradually increasing the pressure. That's the secret, not to start too hard. I would just lie on the bed with my bottom pushed up high by some pillows under my tummy, my skirt flipped up and my knickers around my knees. I'd be really relaxed, just listening to the lovely swishing noise the birch made as it travelled through the air before the explosion of tiny stings scattered across my buttocks, over and over. I like lots of flicks with a riding crop too, and I suppose that was my first experience of corporal punishment, but not my first spanking. I'm not one hundred per cent sure which was the first time, but my first really memorable experience was on a train into Charing Cross from Charlton. I was with my first very dom boyfriend, who's going to have to remain anonymous."

"Okay. You say your first very dominant boyfriend. Do you usually prefer dominant men?"

"I did then. I liked to feel a man wouldn't take any nonsense from me. He was, and still is – we still talk every couple of weeks – very charismatic, strong too, and I'd better make sure I say good-looking or he may pay me a visit! He certainly didn't put up with any of my nonsense, and he'd often threatened to spank me, but I didn't think he'd actually go through with it, let alone the way it happened. Oh, and he liked me to wear short pleated skirts, often ones he'd bought for me, usually tartan school skirts, but some plain or designer styles. He liked me in tight blouses as well, or a tight-fitting polo-neck sweater with no bra, and smart well polished, low-heel leather shoes, sometimes good quality shiny tights, very often no knickers underneath my skirt."

"Sensible man, although I can't agree about the knickers. A girl should always be in knickers, otherwise you miss out on the fun of pulling them down, unless of course that's not going to be an option, in which case yes, no knickers is good. Do go on."

"That's how I was dressed that day, a polo-neck and a pleated mini-skirt with tights underneath, no bra, no knickers. For some reason I'd got it into my head to deliberately annoy him."

"To see if he'd dare to carry out his threat and spank you?"

"Maybe, subconsciously, but it was probably just attention, because he was hardly going to deal with me in such a public place, was he? Or so I thought. Then the last two people besides us in our carriage got out. It was the way he looked at me as the doors closed that made me realise I'd pushed him too far and I was really going to get it, which made me feel scared but excited at the same time. I got up and ran down the carriage, and I really did mean to escape, but he'd realised my intention and was too quick for me. Before I could apologise he grabbed me and threw me across his lap. I got my skirt flipped up and he started to spank me, holding me down, and he was merciless. It really hurt and I thought it couldn't get any worse, but then with one swift movement down went my tights, to my knees. I was bare, but he just didn't care, and as we whizzed past a station he carried on tanning my backside and the backs of legs. I just hope we were going too fast for people to see, but I suspect they did. I tried to kick up my legs to protect myself, but he wrapped one leg across mine and pined me down firmly, making sure I couldn't get away and that if anybody did look in they'd see everything. He spanked me solidly, for ages, while I was begging for mercy. I was trying to apologise too, but he just kept on spanking until I just didn't know what was happening to me. At one point he pushed his finger into my pussy for good measure, and I think he'd have got really dirty with me, only the train was slowing down as it started to pull into the next station. Not that he stopped. We were near the front, and I was well aware that lots of potential passengers on the platform were now getting a flash of my extremely red, upturned bottom. I was struggling desperately, but he was completely unfazed and waited until the train had almost come to a standstill before he threw me onto the opposite seat. He then sat there laughing at my obvious embarrassment as I struggled to pull up my tights. As the doors opened I kept my head down, feeling very flustered and trying to compose myself. Several people got in, and I had to endure the rest of the journey knowing that at least some of people sitting around me had seen me get spanked. Needless to say I was never cheeky to him again, at least not on a train. To this day he still reminds me of the details and finds it extremely amusing."

"And for you?"

"At the time I was too shocked to think about it, except that I was getting a bare-bottom spanking in public, but I have to admit, looking back, I find it a turn-on to think about. It has to go down as one of the most exciting spanking experiences of my life."

Porn in the USA – Erica Scott

I like to think of England as the home of spanking, but there's no doubt our cousins across the pond run us a close second. As far as videos and internet content goes, they're well in the lead, with several outfits producing enough imaginative, high-quality content to keep all but the most particular of spankers happy twenty-fours hours a day. That's not to say our own, home-produced spanking smut is inferior, but the British film classification system makes it almost impossible to operate commercially, with the result that most of the well known internet spanking stars are from the United States. Among them is Erica Scott, famed for her trim figure and delightfully cheeky bottom. Erica is best known for her Shadow Lane Videos, one of which, *Spank Thy Neighbour*, she not only wrote and starred in, but drew from her first spanking experience. A trip to California was a little impractical, but she very kindly sent me a full description of that experience as it happened. Erica –

"My first spanking was probably not your typical spanking, because the man wasn't really a spanker. Nevertheless, I'm extremely grateful to him for the experience, because he was the perfect person for a newbie: sensitive, aware, asked all the right questions, and observed all the proper protocol (which I didn't even know about then). I was thirty-eight years old, seeing someone at the time (vanilla), and it was a casual relationship, both of us free to see others, so I had decided it was time to explore these longtime fantasies. I started answering ads in the Alternatives

141

section of the *LA Weekly* (I had not discovered the Internet yet; I didn't even know how to operate a computer). There were few to none that mentioned spanking, but plenty that mentioned dominance and compliance, and I thought some of those perhaps might include spanking. One ad asked for people who fantasized about being compliant but were too shy to pursue it; claimed he was safe and sane and trustworthy for expressing and exploring one's secrets. Also that he was tall, cute, funny and intelligent, mid-thirties. Perfect, I thought. I called his box number and left a message, and he called me back. We had a brief conversation on the phone. No, he wasn't really experienced in spanking, but it could always be worked into his type of thing. He was more into domination and power play, and very much into elaborate role-playing scenarios. So we agreed to meet for coffee. Remember, at this point I was a total spanking virgin. No experience, no parties, no clue as to what to expect. I even thought I'd end up hating it in reality, even though in fantasy it seemed so delicious.

"So we met; I liked his looks from the start. Very tall, well built, full head of prematurely salt and pepper hair, glasses, clean-shaven, and yes, cute. We had coffee at Starbucks, but decided to take a walk since we didn't want to be overheard. So we talked, and the nervousness and excitement was building. I wanted this. I was scared of this. He seemed pretty laid-back, nonchalant about the whole thing, didn't seem to take it very seriously. He just wanted totally uninvolved exploration, no strings, no emotional ties. His name was Paul, and he asked many questions. What did I want? What did I envision happening? What kind of person was I looking for? What was a typical scene in

142

my fantasies? I told him the best I could, since I really didn't know myself.

"Long story short, after a lot of discussion, we agreed to meet at my apartment the following Monday, which happened to be Memorial Day. The day came. I hadn't been this nervous since the night I lost my virginity. I didn't know what to wear, and I decided on black leggings and a white cropped t-shirt. He showed up, and we had a glass of wine, chatting a bit. Turned out he was a Beatles fan like me, so we made some small talk about that, and then got to the matter of what we'd gotten together for. Had I thought about what kind of scene I wanted to do, he asked. I had done nothing but think about it. I wasn't much good at this role-play business (I'm still not), but I did come up with what I thought was a plausible scenario. We'd be neighbours. I'd be playing my stereo way too loud, and he'd come over to ask me nicely to turn it down. Of course, I'd refuse and be unpleasant about it, and things would take off from there. He asked a lot of questions … would it be OK if he pinned my wrists? Undressed me, or partially undressed me? He said – 'Look, I've never given anyone a spanking before, so I really don't know what's too much or when to stop. Let's choose a safe word and you use it when you've had enough'. So we chose one. He was very thorough, and I look back on that and am so grateful. I mean, I've met people who have been into spanking for years and don't know the concept of safe words.

"Anyway, he walked out the door, and I turned up the stereo. My heart was pounding so hard … was this really going to happen? I mean, after all these years, all this dreaming and planning and fantasizing and wondering and … oh, my God. It was really

143

happening. The knock was at the door, and I was about to answer it in full brat persona. I opened it, and Paul stood there, looking annoyed yet apologetic – 'Hi…look, can you please turn that down a little?'. I snapped back – 'What for, it's only 3:00 in the afternoon'. He said he knew that, but he worked nights and he was trying to sleep now. I said it wasn't my problem that he had such a stupid job, and I couldn't enjoy my music if I turned it down, so he should get some earplugs or get a new job. I started to push the door shut, but he pushed it back open and forced his way past me into the apartment. Then he went over to the stereo and turned the volume down himself. I yelled at him to knock it off, and pushed the volume knob further up than it had been before. He turned it down again. I reached to turn it back up, and he grabbed my wrist. I tried to pull away, told him to let go of me and get out of here, that I don't need this. He grabbed my other wrist and said – 'I know just what you need,' – and he physically dragged me, kicking and struggling and screaming, into the bedroom. He sat on the edge of my bed, pulling me down over one of his legs. My upper half lay across his leg and on to the bed, and my legs hung over the edge. He pulled my leggings down to mid-thigh – I was wearing a thong and that came down too.

"Everything after that is a blur. I remember bits and pieces, like clips from a movie. I remember it hurt a lot, more than I'd imagined it would. I remember I started kicking him, and he said, 'OK, that's enough of that,' and pinned my legs with his other leg. I remember screaming at him, threatening him, swearing at him, thrashing around and fighting like a wild woman, but he was so strong. He had both my wrists pinned in one hand.

"One thing I remember so clearly was his voice. He spoke to me in this calm, very deliberate voice, never raising it. It was almost hypnotic. I'd scream, 'I'm going to get the manager!' and he'd answer, 'No, I don't think you're going anywhere right now'. I'd tell him to stop it, and he'd say, 'Stop? No, we're just getting started here. I think you wanted this all along, didn't you? I'll bet you turned up your music on purpose just so I'd come down here and give you what you need'. For someone who had never given a spanking before, he was doing a damn good job. His dialogue was the type I would have written for a fantasy story.

"It was like having an out-of-body experience – I couldn't believe this was happening to me. And he just kept smacking and smacking and smacking, and talking in that same calm voice … it went on and on. I started saying I was sorry, and, 'OK, I won't tell the manager, I'll keep it down, I promise!' He came right back, 'Sorry? How sorry are you? Nope, I don't think you're quite sorry enough.' He showed no signs of stopping, and then I remembered he'd left it up to me to stop it. But I didn't want to! I really didn't! Somehow, the pain had blurred into something deeply pleasurable, and I found myself wanting more and more. Eventually though, I knew I was making a hell of a lot of noise, and I was concerned about my neighbours hearing and so forth, so I finally yelled out the safe word we'd chosen and he stopped immediately. I lay on the bed, barely able to catch my breath. It was a fairly warm day, and we were both sweating so hard that my comforter on the bed was damp. He got me some water and we lay on the bed side by side for a while, quietly. He didn't say anything, and I didn't know what to say. That was

145

probably the most awkward moment … where does one go from here? I had no clue, and he didn't know either. Instinctively, I wanted to be held and cuddled and soothed, but I didn't know how to ask for it, and I guess he wasn't comfortable doing it. Of course, now I would be horribly put off by a lack of aftercare. But then, I didn't know any better. Aside from that, I don't think he could have done a better job. After a while we both got up and straightened up, and he left shortly thereafter.

"I have no idea what he was thinking after the fact, but I was left on a high that lasted for the rest of the week. I absolutely could not believe that wild, wanton, thrashing woman had been me. There were plenty of after-effects. My throat was raw from all the screaming. Both my wrists were bruised. And the marks on my backside were mesmerizing – you could actually make out a handprint on one cheek. Purple and red streaks everywhere. And yes, I loved every single mark, every bruise. They were my little secrets. I'd gaze at my wrists and smile. I'd go to the gym, dress in the bathroom stall instead of the locker room and smile. I relived the scene, over and over and over again all week and smiled.

"What happened to Paul? He had his own problems; unfortunately, he wanted to keep this part of himself so secret, so apart from the rest of his life, and he told no one – plus he had a vanilla relationship and this double life of his was causing all kinds of guilt. He had thought keeping it totally anonymous would work. I never knew his last name or where he lived, or what he did for work. Plus (and this one hurt) he wasn't all that attracted to me anyway. He assured me it wasn't me, it's just that he had a fetish for a particular type of body – the ultra waifish type, really skinny, like Nicole Richie or Kate Moss. I'm pretty thin, but I'm no waif. Plus, he had a thing for Asian women. So, I didn't see him again. I felt horribly sad and let down for a while, thinking I'd fallen for him, but I soon realized it wasn't him I fell for, but the experience he'd given me. I wanted more, and it was up to me to pursue it. I will never, ever forget him, and will always wish the best for him. Over the years, I have heard many horror stories about women's first scenes with the wrong person, and I think of Paul with gratitude. I hope he is happy and has found what he is looking for. As for me – soon after that I placed my own ad, met my current boyfriend, and the rest is, as they say, history."

The Perils of Journalism – Sarah Berry

Sarah Berry isn't a name you're likely to come across when surfing the net for spanking content, but she deserves her place among the stars. As editor of *Forum Magazine* she ensures that spanking and other kinky delights maintain their position at the heart of the British sex scene, while she herself approaches the subject with unbridled enthusiasm. In the best traditions of investigative journalism she is prepared to try just about anything in the name of research, and when you work for *Forum* that can get very interesting indeed.

I'd heard of Sarah as somebody who was worth knowing quite a while before I met her. She'd been doing her research on assorted kinks and was drawing a great deal of attention. I was intrigued, especially as when it comes to kinky sex most people have strong likes and dislikes but Sarah seemed to be up for anything. That proved to be something of an exaggeration, but not much of one. On meeting Sarah I found her full of energy and imagination, fascinated by all things sexual and yet quite capable of looking after herself. At the time I needed models for a variety of projects, while she needed content for *Forum*, especially records of days out spent indulging exotic kinks. Working together made sense and look like being a lot of fun.

It was. After a little discussion about what she'd like to do and what I was able to offer, we decided that I'd take her out into the deep woods, first for a spot of mud-larking and then for some piggy-girl play. I've seldom packed more fun into one afternoon, from the highly alcoholic picnic lunch to the very end, by which time she was dressed up as an erotic clown in size 12 DMs, bright red knee socks, frilly pink panties and red and white hair ribbons, with her nipples rouged and full face make-up. She was also sporting a huge spanking paddle in one hand and a pair of scotch eggs and an extra large sausage roll in the other. But that's another story. By that point I'd spanked her, using both my hand and a switch cut from the hedge as we walked into the woods, a half-dozen cuts across her perky little bottom while she searched for lemon-scented chocolate truffles among the moss on the forest floor, which is what piggy-girls do, among other things. There was also an incident involving two individual portion chocolate puddings and some highly unusual goings on at a well known motorway service station, but that again is another story. That wasn't so very long after Sarah's first ever spanking, which was taken in the name of research but in a spirit of pure fun. Sarah –

"I'd gone to the Hawthornes Academy to do a piece for *Scarlet Magazine*."

"What is Hawthornes Academy?"

"A sort of pretend school where you go to role-play as an adult schoolgirl. There are several of them, but Hawthornes specialises in girls as pupils and most of the teachers are men."

"And this is the sort of old-fashioned, fantasy school

where bad girls get spanked?"

"Got it in one. I'd never been spanked before, but that was what I was there for, otherwise I wouldn't have been able to do my article properly."

"So a good girl might get away with it?"

"Maybe, but probably not, because if the Headmaster didn't spank her, then her fellow pupils probably would, for being a goody-goody."

"So you go to Hawthornes with the expectation of being spanked?"

"Exactly. I was cheeky from the start, but I didn't get it until I accused Headmaster Jones of sleeping with cabin boys. He called me into his study and told me I was to be spanked. Usually it would have been the cane, but you get to choose how severely you can be punished and I'd gone for just spanking."

"How did it feel to be in that situation, knowing that you'd given him the right to spank you?"

"Pretty real, scary as well as exciting. He's very dominant and my stomach was tying itself in knots at the thought of being put across his knee. He played it for real too, telling me he'd decided on a spanking. Then it was pinafore up and knickers down, bare bottom across his knee. He started to spank me. It was hard and sharp, and I felt genuinely embarrassed to be bare over his knee, mainly because I knew he could see everything and I was sure that he'd notice I was wet."

"So you enjoyed yourself?"

"Oh yes, lots. I'd known I would, because really it's all in the head and I've always liked the idea of submissive sex. It felt best afterwards, when I went to the loo to inspect my rosy cheeks in the mirror. It felt so rude, remembering what he'd done to me and thinking about how he'd seen what I was showing. I imagined it going further, with him getting carried away and making me pose so he could come all over my spanked bottom. I put my hand down the front of my knickers and finished myself off, watching."

"Very nice."

"It was, and that wasn't the end of it. I knew I could take more. I was high in a way I'd never been before, high on spanking. I went back into the classroom and carried on being cheeky until he pulled me up and spanked me in front of the whole class."

"Knickers down?"

"Oh yes. It's always knickers down."

"Just as it should be. And it was obviously a good introduction as now you enjoy regular spankings?"

"Yes, but with me it is very much spanking, although I have tried implements. At one Night of the Cane I went into the competition, but it was too much. It's all rather impersonal as well. I much prefer skin on skin contact, and when you're over a man's knee there's always the chance of an erection to squirm on."

"I bet there is!"

The Anonymous Star – ? ?

I wasn't at all sure where to put this one, or whether to put it in at all. The young lady in question was absolutely insistent that she remain completely nameless and also that I give no hint whatsoever as to her true identity. I am therefore unable to explain our background or give away more than that her name would be immediately recognisable to any dedicated spanking enthusiast. Nor am I permitted to describe her, again for fear of giving away her identity. I am allowed to give the full details of her first spanking, for the simple reason that the version she has given in interviews and put in print is a fantasy. This is the reality, too peculiar and too embarrassing for her to admit to openly. A star –

"I got into the spanking scene as soon as I could. All I wanted was a partner who would give me the regular discipline I craved and let me play, a sugar daddy I suppose, but the money was too easy to resist. I attended my first spanking party at eighteen, and did my first video. You've got to see it from my point of view. I was only a student but I could afford my own flat, more or less anything I wanted too. There was nobody to control me, because I was getting all the discipline I wanted ... no, that I needed, and still do need, but I'd realised that one man wasn't enough and I couldn't find a man who'd put up with my lifestyle. I chose the lifestyle."

"I don't suppose you could find a man who could afford to keep you either, by the sound of it?"

"There were offers, believe me, but in the end they always wanted me under their thumb. It's ironic. I always wanted to be protected but I've always had to fight."

"And you won, I'd say."

"I'm all right, that's true. At the time it was all just one thing after another, parties and videos and clubs, and spankings, all the spankings I needed, and the more I got the more I craved it. My flat was full of gear, every sort of spanking implement you can think of, and clothes, and rope, and spanking magazines, lots of spanking magazines. I love them. I only have to open one of my favourite issues of *Kane* or *Blushes* and I want to get the same as the girls inside are getting, even when I've just had it. Which has to do with how I got my first, because I had the magazines before I got into the spanking scene.

"You've got to understand, spanking is like a drug to me. I had three magazines, that's all, at first. I used to take them with me, wherever I went, my secret thrill. I

151

knew every single picture and every single story. When I went down to my grandparents' place in ----- I'd take them, and that was where I went wrong. Basically, Gran found one of the magazines. She was furious. She really went on about it, telling me how wrong-headed I was – that was her favourite expression, wrong-headed. She used to use it for anything she didn't agree with – and how stupid I was, letting myself think something so perverted was exciting. No, not perverted. 'Unfortunate' – that's the word she used, as if me being spanked was something that might be necessary, but if it was it would be a serious matter, not something … something playful, and definitely not sexual! "

"So she realised you were getting off on the magazines?"

"Oh yes. She wasn't stupid. She knew exactly what I was up to. She knew an awful lot, actually, thinking about it, but she definitely didn't approve. She told me she was going to teach me a lesson, show me that it wasn't funny, or exiting, that it was thoroughly nasty – her exact words – 'thoroughly nasty' – she said. Up until then I'd just stood there like an idiot, looking at my feet and feeling sorry for myself and, I don't know, I just did as I was told, I suppose, or rather, I didn't stop her. I don't know why, but I didn't even protest, not properly, even when she actually said she was going to spank me. Imagine it, me standing there like a complete idiot while she turned up my dress at the back and made me hold it, then pulled down my knickers. That's how she spanked me, smacking my bum and telling me off. I felt so stupid, and so small, standing there, holding my own skirt up with my knickers round my knees while she spanked me! She did it really hard too, as hard as she could, and she kept going on about how she'd show me it hurt and it wasn't nice at all. The trouble was, it was lovely. Not then, not while she was doing it. That just felt weird, and seriously embarrassing, but once she'd finished and stormed off out of the room I was just left there, still with my knickers down, just in a daze. It had only taken a couple of minutes, but it was like a gigantic shock. All I could think about was that I'd been spanked, for the first time in my life you understand. I went on to the bed and just lay there, on my side at first and then on my tummy. I couldn't bring myself to cover up, not even to pull up my knickers. It just felt right like that, bare, with my dress right up round my waist and my knickers round my knees. I thought she'd come back, at first, but after a bit I could hear her clattering around downstairs, making the tea. I just had to do it. I started to touch my hot bum and that really brought it home. There I was, knickers down on the bed, my bum all hot from spanking. My cheeks felt hot and big, like they were my centre. I couldn't stop touching. I couldn't face the reality, that Gran had spanked me in order to show me how nasty it was. That was just funny, in a weird way, because I'd never been so turned on. I had to touch myself off. I don't mean I wanted to. I had to, like that, face down on the bed with my spanked bum pushed up and my hand between my legs. I even pulled up my knickers a bit, just so I could hold them and know they'd been pulled down, but in my head it was a man who'd done it, and he'd done it because I needed to be spanked. I still do, and maybe two hundred different men must have spanked me – you get forty at some parties – but I still need spanking and I still haven't found the right man."

With the interview complete I couldn't help but point out that she came across as a bit of a brat. She laughed.

Turning the Tables – spankings for dominant women

OLD-SCHOOL THOUGHT ON kinky behaviour divides people firmly and irrevocably into two categories: those who like to dish it out – the dominant, the sadist – and those who like to take it – the submissive, the masochist. Why this should be I have no idea, when the great majority of people prefer a bit of each, making them what's called a switch. Even de Sade was a switch. Nevertheless, so deeply ingrained is this idea, and so strong the desire of many submissive men for a stern, unyieldingly dominant mistress that a great many women who are dominant at heart but enjoy a little variety only express their submissive side in private, or with a few select partners. For me, the idea of a dominant woman accepting a spanking exerts a particular fascination, especially if it's her first time. That's a rare privilege, but all the sweeter for that, and I made a special effort to record the first spanking experiences of women who are naturally dominant and seldom show their more yielding side.

Unfairly Beaten – Pippa Green

Most people on the fetish scene address Pippa as Mistress, and she looks and acts the part. Tall, assertive and well built, she is one of those women who dominate a situation simply by being there. Sexual submission is a state of mind, but with Pippa you know that once you're in position over her knee it's not simply that you don't want to get up, but that you can't get up. That appeals to a lot of men, and women too, and Pippa takes a particular pleasure in rising to the challenge. Pippa –

"I love to wrestle, and I love to win. Nearly always I do, and that not just the subby guys who want to lose anyway. That's not so much fun, which is why I prefer to play with switches, 'cause with a switch I know I have to win, for real, or I'm going to be the one who gets her bum smacked, and believe me, that's far more humiliating for me than it is for most people."

"I can see that, but I bet it doesn't happen very often?"

"No, not very often, never with another woman and not with many men. You cheated."

What I actually did was decline to wait until I'd won, or she'd won, but instead got a good grip on the waistband of her panties, pulled them up as tight as they would go and spanked her like that, with most of her weight lifted clear of the floor by a thin strip of cotton tugged up between her pussy lips. I like to think of that as good tactics. She says it's cheating. What I didn't know at the time was that it was the first time she'd ever been spanked. Twice before she'd been taken to the edge but given the option of crying off, and she hadn't expected me to take it as part and parcel of wrestling together. Pippa –

"You just did it! I didn't realise that's what you were up to, even when you gave me the wedgie, and then you'd started to spank me and it was too late. Can you imagine how that felt, all those years and never been spanked and then you come along and just lay in! I always knew it might happen eventually, but I expected it to be a big deal, you know, with a lot of ceremony about me dressing the right way, and being prepared, and being told what I was going to get, and all that, not just wedgied and smacked on the floor like it was no big deal at all!"

"You'd have done the same to me."

"No. I'd have made you submit and accept your spanking."

"But both times somebody made you submit you used your safe word."

'I know. I just couldn't go through with it. It felt too humiliating, but you just went ahead and did it, and once I was being spanked, that was it. It was too late."

"You made a hell of a fuss over it."

"It hurt! You didn't expect me to give in, did you? One thing I'm not is submissive."

"But you didn't use your safe word, did you?"

"No. It didn't occur to me at first. I was just too shocked at what you were doing, and, I don't know, since I was being spanked anyway I felt I might as well let you get on with it, because you were obviously enjoying yourself so much."

"That's true. I only wish I'd known it was your first time while I was doing it, because I'd have enjoyed that even more. The way you reacted I assumed you'd had it many a time."

"How do you mean?"

"You were playing with yourself, Pippa. You came while I was spanking you. That's not how first-timers usually behave, is it?"

"Okay, okay, so I'm not submissive, I'm really not, but I am a masochist, when the situation is right. You were spanking me. You had my knickers right up tight. You seemed to think it was just a laugh, but for me it was really important. I wanted it to be special, something I'd remember for ever."

'And was it?"

'Oh yes! And thank you very much for not stopping until I'd come."

From her Best Friend's Daughter – Natalie Parr

Natalie wasn't spanked until she was in her early forties, although it had always been a fantasy for her. I met her when we were first involved with the fetish scene and she was already an established player. More dominant than otherwise, she spanked me before I spanked her, a dose of the riding crop while bent across a table in a bar hired for the night by a club called Café Ensemble. I had my revenge in a matter of minutes, after a few more glasses of wine had loosened her resolve, and that in itself was something of a first, for me. Never before had I spanked a woman who was older then me, but at the time I had no idea how important that was for her, or why. Had I been older than her she would almost certainly have turned me down. This is why.

She was dominant to her partner, who was also present, and in a club full of adoring men who wanted nothing more than to taste the sting of her crop or kiss her booted feet. What they did not want, or expect, was to see her skin-tight black leather dress rolled up to her waist, her lacy black knickers pulled down and her bare bottom smacked to a glowing pink. That was what she got from me, bent across the same table and done in front of a good half-dozen of her admirers, and the reason she allowed it to happen was that I had unwittingly tapped into one of her strongest fantasies. Had I been younger still, and female, the situation would have been perfect.

To fully appreciate her fantasy and the strength of her first ever spanking we need to go back a bit. Natalie is tall, elegant and blessed with a smile that seems to be forever hinting at mischief. Her accent is distinctly upper-class and she has never lost the poise instilled at the all-girls boarding school she attended from the 50s until she left at the age of sixteen. On the fetish scene that makes her the classic English dominatrix, which is a genuine reflection of her sexuality, but not the whole story. On the wall of her flat is a photograph taken towards the end of the 60s. It looks as if it might have come from the cover of a pop album. From the smart, dark bob of her hair to the long, long legs that stretch down from the hem of her microdress she is every inch a hippy-chick, soft and feminine but also rebellious and with just a touch of youthful, privileged arrogance, in fact, just the sort of girl you might feel would deserve a good spanking.

She felt she did, but only in her darkest, most private moments. Otherwise it was unthinkable, not only anathema to everything she believed in but directly opposed to the main thrust of her sexuality, how she saw herself and how others saw her. In her own words –

"I was married at twenty and my husband worshipped me. I was his rebel girl, but we were from the same background so it was perfect, or it should have been. You have to remember that what we look back to as the lifestyle of the 60s was only true for a handful of people, mostly in London and mostly well off. I was one of them, but only because we lived in South Kensington and could afford to keep up with fashion. David was a farmer's son from Lincolnshire. He was big and handsome, so I was flattered, I suppose, but there was always a contradiction in the way he behaved towards me. He was always saying how he admired me for being strong-willed and independent, but he treated me like bone china. Sex was good, at least at first. He loved me to go on top and to generally take control. Looking back I realise he had a submissive sexuality, but that wouldn't have meant anything to me at the time, or to him either. It was

158

just the way we liked it, and it was how I felt it should be. Only just occasionally I'd get this nagging little urged to be treated a little rough, to be taken in hand and made to please him, and above all to be spanked. I never admitted it to him. I could hardly bear to admit it to myself!"

"But you used to fantasise?"

"Yes, but it was a guilty pleasure."

"Tell me."

"If I must. At first I used to wish David would do it. He's six foot four and he'd worked on the land all his life, so you can imagine how strong he was as a young man. He has huge hands, and I used to imagine how they'd feel on my bottom, not just cupping my cheeks the way he used to, but spanking me. He could have done it so easily, just put me across his lap and spanked me. I used to imagine how it would feel, how angry I'd be and how helpless, how he wouldn't pay any attention to my protests but just carry on in the same methodical fashion he brought to everything else, lifting up my skirt and slip, pulling down my knickers and spanking my bare bottom."

"And you always used to imagine yourself bare?"

"Doesn't everybody?"

"Most people, certainly. But you said you only wished David would do it at first?"

"Yes. After a while I realised that he just wasn't right, and he was my husband, which somehow ..."

"Took the edge off the fantasy?"

"Yes. That's it, exactly. It felt stronger if I imagined a stranger doing it, or one of the farmhands, even one of their wives, which made me so guilty I cried afterwards."

"After you'd come?"

"Yes, but it was amazing, different to when I was with

David, maybe better. After that I'd do anything to make it stronger."

"More embarrassing?"

"Yes, I suppose so, but more than that, anything to make me feel I was being brought down, put in my place, anything inappropriate."

Natalie's marriage lasted nearly eighteen years and she never did get spanked. In fact she was the model of a respectable country wife, involved with the parish and local affairs, the perfect helpmeet to her husband and the perfect mother to her two sons. Yet before too long she had begun to feel that life was passing her by and when her husband was caught out in an affair with a local wife she left him and moved back to London. She had never lost contact with her old friends and ended up staying with a girl she'd been to school with, Cordelia, who had also married young and was now divorced. This was the end of the 80s and they would sometimes meet up in a Soho pub where Cordelia's daughter worked behind the bar to help support herself though university. Natalie –

"I was fascinated by Gemma from the start. She was so like I had been at that age, self-assured, confident of where she was going, determined, only where I'd always imagined myself getting married she was set on a career as well. There was also something faintly mocking about the way she treated her mother, and myself as one of her mother's friends, as if there was something comic about us."

"That must have been annoying, but I suppose it's not an unusual attitude from a young woman to her mother?"

"I suppose not, and it was annoying, although they got on well enough most of the time, and so did we. Gemma and myself that is."

160

"I know Gemma, so I can guess what's coming."

"Yes, the little bitch! She says she saw it in my eyes the first time we met, but I don't believe her."

"But she must have guessed."

"Not at first, I don't think. She used to go out a lot, and sometimes she'd dress outrageously, in black leather mostly, and not much of it, and having blazing rows with Cordelia. She was going to Submission and Torture Garden, which had just started, but I thought she was working in a strip joint or something like that. She'd come back very late and on such a high I thought she'd been taking drugs. She'd be very assertive as well, even towards her mother."

"But you didn't realise what she was into?"

"No. I was naive, I suppose. I just thought she was exceptionally self-assured, and a bit of a brat."

"So how did it happen?"

"Cordelia and I had started to date again. We'd always go out together, but this time she met a man she really liked. At the end of the evening she asked if I'd mind if she stayed over with him, and so I ended up going back to the flat alone. I was feeling a bit sorry for myself, I suppose, and I'd already had quite a bit to drink, so I opened myself a bottle of wine and put Ruthless People on the video. I'd drunk most of the bottle and I was right at the end of the film when Gemma came back. She called out to ask if her mother was back but I told her it was me. She began to talk as she took her coat off, then from the kitchen, so I told her to hush because I was right at the end of the film. She did, but she came in a couple of minutes later, just as I was taking the cassette out of the recorder, kneeling down. She was in one of her outfits, boots and shorts over fishnets and a leather waistcoat with nothing underneath. She had a riding

161

whip in one hand and a peanut butter sandwich in the other."

"Not quite the perfect dominant image. And what were you wearing?"

"Tight black jeans. Looking back I suppose that when you're used to it and somebody's got their bum stuck out, you smack it, especially after several hours at a club. She only patted my bottom with the riding whip and told me not to tell her to be quiet, that's all, and really it shouldn't have been important. It didn't hurt, but that's not what matters. I reacted. I couldn't stop myself. I was angry, but only slightly and only for a moment, and then I'd started to blush. I tried to hide it but that only made it worse. She told me to look at her and I tried to tell her off but she started to laugh, and then she said it."

"What?"

"'Oh my, Nutty Natalie likes to be spanked!' Her exact words. I could have screamed. I should have kept calm, telling her to go up to her room and sleep it off, because she was as drunk as I was. Instead I tried to deny it, but she only laughed at me, then sat down on the sofa, grinning. I'd never been so embarrassed in my life. I didn't know what to do and I didn't know what to say. She didn't seem to care, but took a bite of her sandwich and a swallow from my bottle of wine then lay back, stretching herself out. I had to say something to deny it, because I was sure she'd tell her mother, but when I came over to her she just looked up at me, smiling. Maybe she misread my intentions. She says it was what I wanted all along, but she spoke first and I remember every word – 'Go on then, stick it out. I don't mind doing you'."

"And she spanked you?"

"No, not then. I wish I'd let her. That way I could at least look as if I handled it well! I didn't. I ran up to my room, as if I was about six and my mum had caught me with my hands in the biscuit box. It came about six weeks later. We both knew, and I suppose it was only a matter of time. She kept teasing me, and giving me little pats if she caught me alone. I'd tell her to stop it, to show me some respect, but she'd just laugh and respond that if it was what I wanted I should let her do it. In the end it was me who asked for it. Every night the same thoughts had been going through my head, about how good it would be to let her have her way, just once, and that would be enough. For some reason I also imagined that she'd dress up and use her riding whip on me, which would have made it easier to take, less personal I suppose. What happened was very different. She did me OTK, sitting on the end of her mother's bed, and okay she'd already given me quite a few pats, but that was my first spanking, my first real spanking."

"Do you mind going into a bit more detail?"

"I suppose not. I'd been telling myself I'd let her do it, just once, but in the end I had to ask for it. That was right, because it added to the embarrassment, but that was nothing to how I felt about her being the one to do it. You understand, so you'll know how I felt as I got down across her lap, but from another woman, half my age and worst of all, my best friend's daughter! I just had to have it, but for all her experience she was much less mature than I was, than I am, so instead of being understanding about my desires she was an absolute bitch. First she made me ask for it a second time, out loud, standing in front of her in her room and actually saying the words – 'Please, Gemma, I'd like you to spank me' – and then

163

she took me into her mother's bedroom. Cordelia was out, but she might have come back at any time and I kept having visions of her catching me across her daughter's knee with a red bottom. Gemma knew, but she didn't seem to care, telling me to take down my jeans in front of her, then to bend over her lap. I was almost crying with frustration and shame, but I wanted to do it so badly I couldn't stop myself. To be across her knee was the worst thing that had ever happened to me and the best, all at the same time. I felt utterly ashamed of myself but it was bliss at the same time. I was shaking and right on the edge of tears, but she was determined to push it. She made me pull up my top and bra, telling me it was a necessary part of the punishment to have my breasts bare, and she had a good feel. Then it was my bottom. No ceremony, the way I'd always imagined it in my fantasies, just knickers down as if it was completely unimportant, as if laying my bottom bare for spanking was just one of those things, like taking a coat off when you come indoors. Then she spanked me."

"Tell me."

"It was hard, and it hurt. For the first few smacks I was thinking that I must have been completely mad to ever want anything of the sort. I tried to get up, but she'd been expecting that and twisted my arm behind my back, which didn't stop me struggling or begging her to stop. That was what finally made her realise that I couldn't cope the way she seemed to expect me to. She told me it would be all right, just that, and I honestly think that if she hadn't said those words I'd have made it stop and maybe never gone back to it. There is something amazing about being soothed by the person who's spanking you though, and she'd stopped doing it so hard and begun to stroke my bottom between smacks. I just gave in. It was too nice to resist, everything I'd ever imagined and far more. She carried on for ages, smacking and stroking my cheeks, calling me a bad girl and even telling me how funny it would be if her mother came in and caught her spanking me. In no time she had me in a sort of haze of pleasure, what they call subspace now. I wanted it to go on for ever, and hard, for all that it hurt. I'd never felt so humiliated in my life, bare over a twenty-year-old's knee with everything showing and my bottom growing pink to the slaps as she laughed at me and told me how comic I looked. Every word stung, and I was thinking over and over of how I was being spanked by my best friend's daughter, but it was ecstasy, the kind of ecstasy I'd only ever imagined before. Things have changed and I don't often show my submissive side nowadays, but if there's one thing that can really get to me it's being spanked by somebody younger than I am and in especially embarrassing circumstances."

"So that was your first time. Wonderful. One last question: did you come?"

"You don't want much, do you? No, not while she was doing it. I never do. Afterwards, yes, while I thought about what had happened, and not just the once, maybe a hundred times."

Nearly twenty years separate Natalie's first spanking from the present, but she's never lost her enjoyment of having the tables turned on her, seldom spanked but deeply appreciative when it does happen. She and Gemma have been friends all that time, and while I've watched them work together on men many a time and once or twice been privileged to watch them play with each I never knew that it was Gemma who'd given Natalie her first spanking, nor that it had been such a powerful and important experience.

Even a Goddess needs Spanking – Gemma Clark

Gemma's spanking story follows on in natural sequence from Natalie's and is also similar in that both women are sexually dominant but with a submissive streak. In Natalie's case she is open about that side of her sexuality, but with Gemma it is very carefully hidden. For many years I assumed she was that rare thing, a completely, naturally dominant woman. To read the literature, watch the movies, even surf the web, you might think unleavened sexual dominance was common among women, even the norm, but in practise that is more a reflection of submissive male desire than reality. In just the same way the idea that all outwardly sexually dominant women have a hidden submissive side is a reflection of dominant male desire, and in practise almost everybody, male or female and all but the most straight-laced have at least a little of each desire. Gemma certainly has, but you wouldn't know it to meet her, even at a fetish club. I've changed her name by request, along with one or two other details.

Anybody critical of fetishism, sadomasochistic sex and so forth might argue that Gemma was groomed. Certainly she was introduced to the London fetish scene by an older man, and she was admittedly young, although very much an adult and capable of making her own decisions. I prefer to think of her as a natural, and she certainly took to it, like a duck to water. By her early twenties she was a regular at London's fetish clubs; Submission, Torture Garden and later Club Whiplash, which simply wouldn't have been the same without her. After a couple of years and numerous offers she turned professional and has remained so, despite now being married.

I met her when Penny and I first came onto the fetish

scene, and it was obvious that we were unlikely ever to play together. At the time she believed in female sexual supremacy, the idea that women are naturally superior and dominant to men, which had been instilled into her by her older, submissive partner of the time. In practice she was still finding herself, and watching her at those early clubs it was quite obvious she much preferred to play with other women. That meant we had a lot of playmates in common, so while I didn't know her particularly well we did know a lot about each other.

In appearance Gemma is the classic dominatrix, tall, slender, toned, with long legs and high, firm bottom cheeks, perhaps a little too tight and muscular for my personal taste but sufficiently round and feminine to excite my interest. Besides, there's something about an openly dominant woman that brings out a wicked streak in me. I always wanted to spank her, and while a cynic might argue that it would be quite difficult to find a woman I didn't want to spank, in Gemma's case the idea went beyond simple physical appeal or an expression of sadism. She was forbidden fruit, which is always the sweetest.

Not that I had any intention of doing anything about my desire. I'd heard her say that she had never submitted to anybody and never would so often it was as if it was her personal mantra. That same mantra was repeated by her male slaves and clients with tedious frequency. To them it was clearly important that she be untouchable, which made me want to spank her all the more. It had occurred to me that perhaps she protested a little too much, but I put that down to my own wishful thinking. What I was absolutely certain of was that it was pointless to approach her at a club, because whatever her more private feelings she was definitely not going to accept a trip across my knee in public. There was good reason for that, and there still is. Gemma, after her spanking –

"For a lot of my gentlemen it's really important to believe in me as totally dominant. If they ever found out what you just did to me it would totally destroy their image of me. They wouldn't come back."

I can see her point. After all, if you worship a woman as the physical incarnation of a Goddess you really don't want to see her bent across another man's knee with her bare red bum stuck up in the air and a vibrator up her pussy. It's sacrilege. I rather like committing sacrilege.

In fact, Gemma had been nursing a desire to be spanked for several years. Not from the very start, but as she gathered more and more submissive female playmates who openly enjoyed being spanked she grew curious. She also understood the physical pleasure of spanking, a matter of nerves and hormones that has nothing to do with dominance and submission, and with time came to realise that the idea of one sex being inherently superior to the other is absurd. More than ten years after she had first applied a whip to a man's buttocks she finally asked Nikki, her closest friend and playmate, to spank her, only to find that Nikki didn't want to. Nikki didn't feel right about it, and for similar but more complicated reasons to those of so many of Gemma's clients. Unlike Gemma's clients, Nikki didn't object to the thought of her friend getting it from somebody else. In fact the idea rather appealed. Nikki was also a close friend of ours and suggested that I should be the one to spank Gemma. That didn't go down well at all and there the matter rested for another year.

As far as I remember I didn't see Gemma for a long while after that, but we were then thrown into each other's company. Nikki was getting married, and doing it in style, a church wedding with all the trimmings. Gemma was to be maid of honour and I was chief usher. That meant lots of meetings, but some of the people involved, including the couple's parents, had no idea what they were into and so we always had to be very careful about what was said. It's amusing and feels more than a little strange to be chivvied out of a room by a proud and anxious mother because she wants to discuss the more intimate details of her daughter's wedding finery when you and the prospective groom have had that same sweet, girl strapped near-naked across a whipping bench the night before. You feel that you're part of some clandestine and wicked society, which you are, at least informally. Not being able to discuss our mutual interests certainly helped create a strong sense of camaraderie, and as I drove Gemma back across London after maybe the third or fourth meeting we were getting on better than we ever had before. Nevertheless, when she asked if I'd like to come in for coffee I had no idea she would end up over my knee. I wouldn't have asked.

She did. After two hours of quite intense and increasingly intimate conversation she told me what Nikki had suggested. There was a husky note to her voice and it was obvious she wanted it and out of more than mere curiosity. Yet we still had a way to go, and it took another half-hour of gentle persuasion, of joking and teasing, of bargaining and negotiation before I finally took her down across my knee. The next few minutes were pure bliss. I take immense pleasure in dishing out a spanking to any woman, but to have Gemma was as if I'd been admiring the display in the window of a merchant of fine wines and the proprietor had come out to offer me a free bottle of Château Lafite.

Part of our agreement was that I should treat her no differently to any other girl, and so I allowed myself free rein as I got her into spanking position, anticipating the thought of what I was about to do and how she would look with her bottom bare. Gemma –

"You have no idea how I felt the way you put me, almost upside down, with my head dangling down like that and my bum the highest part of my body. I'd

169

done it to other people so many times, and I kept thinking of the last time I'd sat on my couch, with one guy serving me drinks and nibbles in a maid's outfit and another kneeling down so I could use him as a footstool. If they'd seen me!"

"I would love to have done it in front of them."

"I know you would, you bastard!"

In fact they would have been a distraction, and I wanted to concentrate on what I was doing. She was in a dress, Laura Ashley I think, because the whole wedding business was all very smart. I turned it up, deliberately slowly, to find that she had a slip underneath. That followed, revealing stockings clipped up with a suspender belt so that the flesh of her thighs bulged a little around the straps, and then her bottom, in pretty white panties that were mostly lace at the back and not only hugged her cheeks to perfection but hinted at the glories of what was beneath. I left her like that for a while and turned my attention to her top half. She's quite busty, and I'd always wanted to touch her breasts, so I unzipped the back of her dress and pulled up her bra, leaving them hanging down among dishevelled material, each a plump handful of flesh, surprisingly heavy and tipped by a large, stiff nipple. I played with them for a bit, until she'd begun to moan with pleasure, then turned my attention back to her bottom. Gemma –

"I remember what you said – 'Think of all the people you've done this to. Now it's your turn.' I almost got up."

She didn't, but I could feel her shaking as I peeled those big, lacy knickers slowly down over her cheeks. I like to get a girl fully bare, so that everything's showing from behind and she knows it, but lowered panties do look sweet, so I settled them around her knees and gave her a little smack on the inside of each thigh to make her part her legs and pull the material taut. I had to do it twice, and remind her that she'd asked to be made to do as she was told, but her thighs came open in the end. I cocked my knee up, to lift her bottom and make her brace her feet on the floor, which left her cheeks open as well as her thighs. Her bottom hole was showing and her pussy. I told her, even though she was shaking so badly I was worried that it might be too much for her. She'd begun to sob, but some girls like to cry and she didn't try and get up, so I counted to ten in my head to let the position she was in really sink in and then began to spank her.

I knew it would probably be my only chance, so I really went to town with her, gently at first, because you should never go in too hard, especially with a girl who's not used to it. In between spanks I explored her body, her breasts as well as her bottom. She didn't seem to mind, for all that her reactions were extraordinarily strong, shaking badly and gulping in air as if she'd just come up from under water. I was expecting her to say she'd had enough at any moment, but she stayed put, encouraging me to spank a little harder and take even more liberties, tweaking her nipples and cupping her pussy in my hand. Soon her bottom was nicely flushed, a rich, even pink across both cheeks, while there was no mistaking the scent of female arousal in the air or the way the mouth of her vagina had begun to bead with juice.

If I remember rightly I apologised as I slid my finger up her, because I had said I wouldn't get too dirty with her. She responded with a deep moan and stuck her bottom up, and that was the end of my restraint. I began to spank her hard, fingering her at the same time, then slipping my hand under her pussy to masturbate her, determined to make her come while she was spanked. She was there in no time at all, wriggling her bottom against my hand in the lewdest manner imaginable and begging me to do it harder. I obliged, and while I was turned on that was not my over-riding emotion. That was triumph, to have the cool, dominant Gemma, a

171

Goddess to so many men, writhing and squirming across my lap, boobs and bottom naked, letting me spank her and masturbate her at the same time, and not so much for my pleasure as for her ecstasy.

Then there was the final, perfect touch. Part of our agreement was that once I'd spanked her she would restore her affronted dignity by taking me into her dungeon and doing whatever she wanted. She took me in her mouth instead, on her knees in front of me, happily sucking cock.

Fixated on her Bottom – Kirsten

Kirsten works as a high-class call-girl with a sideline in domination. It was never really her thing, but she looks the part – nearly six foot tall in her stockinged feet, slender, with extraordinarily long legs and ash blonde hair framing a handsome, slightly severe face. Not surprisingly many of her clients wanted her to dominate them, and while she was happy to oblige she had no idea what to do. So she began to learn, visiting clubs and fetish markets, which was where I met her while I was giving a demonstration of different corporal punishment techniques. By then she was experienced but still keen to learn and, unlike many professional dominas, quite happy to switch roles. We played for a while, testing old fashioned implements on each other, first a long-handled shoe horn, then a carpet beater and lastly a horsehair flywhisk, but it was because her bottom was infinitely more lovely than my own that she ended up over my knee for a knickers-down spanking before telling me the story of her first time. Kirsten –

> "It was only a few months ago, when I'd just started out on my learning curve. A friend of mine I sometimes did doubles with knew a transvestite called Joanna who's an expert in corporal punishment …"

"This is honey blonde, TV Joanna, I expect? She gets everywhere."

"I suppose so. She was really good to me, anyhow. She took me around London, buying stuff and showing me how not to get ripped off, like getting riding whips from a horsey place instead of a fetish supplier, and she let me experiment on her, showing me how a man's body reacts to pain, and how to beat somebody. Like you said just now, you can't really appreciate it unless you try it yourself, so I let her, first with her hand and then with different implements, even a cane."

"May I have little more detail please?"

"How do you … oh, I see what you want. We'd gone back to her house after a shopping trip. One of my clients wanted me to dress in a rubber cat suit and had agreed to pay for the whole outfit, in advance. That was some shopping trip. I'd got the suit, in skin-tight black rubber with a hood that leaves just my face showing and my hair sticking up from the top in a ponytail, rubber gloves too, and knee-length boots, all in shiny black. I've always had a fixation on my bottom, and I was showing off to myself in the mirror, looking at the way the rubber covered my cheeks but showed off every single tiny detail, around my pussy lips too. Joanna seemed to like it and I let her touch, which was the first time between us. We'd already talked about how I ought to learn how it felt to be beaten, but I hadn't said she could. She asked, with one hand on my bum, in this surprisingly firm voice … firm but gentle too, and I just didn't feel able to refuse. She began to smack me, very gently, and I don't know, but I just took to it straight away. It looked … sexy, and it made me feel like I wanted sex. It's hard to describe, especially to a man, but if you

173

stroke a female cat when she's on heat she'll stick her bottom up. It made me feel like that, every little pat making me want to stick my bum out a little more, until I was doing it, and still watching in the mirror, with little ripples spreading out across my rubbery black cheeks as Joanna's smacks got gradually harder."

"That sounds like her technique."

"She can be very persuasive, Joanna, and she can be a sneaky bitch. She carried on until my whole bum was warm with this lovely rosy glow, then asked if she could show me how some of the implements felt. I said she could and she immediately pointed out that it would be a shame to damage my brand new cat-suit, especially as I was supposed to wear it for the first time for my client. So off came my cat-suit, and of course that meant taking off my gloves and boots too, so she had me naked and horny, too horny to care. Not just that though. She felt safe, like I was safe in her hands. So I got down on the sofa and stuck out my bottom for her, with my knees right apart. She started to use the implements, telling me about each one, how hard to use it and why leather and wood feel different, everything. She has one of everything too, even a genuine old carpet beater like yours, which she says she got from her aunt, and several paddles, and different whips, and lots of different canes. She used them all, just about, one after another and never too hard, until I was so wet I was ready for anything. It was only when she made me get up and inspect my bare bum in the mirror that I realised I was quite badly marked, far worse than I'd have ever imagined I could take, but it just felt lovely.

"She ordered me to kneel on the sofa again, in that same firm way, only this time she started to massage me and play with my pussy. I'd never been so turned on, and it was far, far better than anything I've experienced with a boyfriend, let alone a client. She took me all the way, without ever once expecting anything in return, and it wasn't until I'd finished that I realised she had the most enormous erection sticking up under the little skirt she'd put on when we dressed up. So I said thank you, the best way I know."

"Which is?"

Kirsten didn't answer, but opened her mouth to make a soft, wet hole rimmed by scarlet lipstick with the tip of a sharp pink tongue just visible inside her mouth. It was getting very difficult to concentrate, especially with the couple on the next settee along in the chill out room where I was interviewing Kirsten. The girl was moaning, eyes closed and legs spread as her boyfriend tugged at her tightly clamped nipples and rubbed the front of her wet black panties. Kirsten glanced at them and smiled, then once more pursed her lips into an inviting O, this time clearly for my benefit. She went on –

"I do like to say thank you for a spanking."

"Well, yes. And you say you prefer being spanked to doing the spanking, and domination in general?"

"Yes. Joanna brought something out in me I hadn't realised was there. I was always fixated on my bottom, but she'd showed me just how much fun that could be. I love any attention, but spanking best of all. I suppose you could say she made me realise the full potential of my bottom. I only do it for fun though, never professionally. That would spoil it for me. I've been out to lots of clubs – with Joanna once, both dressed as schoolgirls – and I've had quite a few offers, of film work too, but I only take money for domme work. It's not so special."

"I think you're very sensible. I've known too many girls who grew jaded, or just lost their taste for spanking because of the dynamics of pro-work. That's great, thanks."

"Is there anything else?"

"You could always say thank you for that spanking, otherwise I think the journey home on the tube could be highly embarrassing. Oh, and if you could pass my address on to Joanna. I'm determined to interview her."

The Ones That Got Away – friends who've been spanked, but not by me

MY EXPERIENCE IS THAT if a girl likes me enough to enjoy sexual contact she'll at least accept a spanking, and more often than not enjoy a spanking. Inevitably there are exceptions, for whatever reason, and among those exceptions there are girls who I'd dearly like to have spanked, who enjoy spanking, but for one reason or another have managed to escape feeling the sting of my hand across their rear cheeks. Here then are three that got away.

Shame in the Sun – Katie Peters

Katie Peters was first spanked on the beach at a well known south coast resort. I know, because she told me afterwards, her face pink with embarrassment and excitement and her bottom much the same colour. All she had on was a short, loose dress over a miniscule, bright red bikini. She pulled the dress up to show me, all the while complaining bitterly about her boyfriend's treatment of her rear cheeks. I tried to be sympathetic, but I was wishing it had been me who'd spanked her and she knew it. She'd also enjoyed it, although that doesn't mean her embarrassment was any less genuine, and we'll come to that later.

Ours was an odd relationship. She knew I was into spanking, because she was a friend of Debbie, and while she used to call me a pervert to my face it was obvious that the idea fascinated her. Whenever she had the opportunity she

177

would bring the subject up, deliberately tormenting me until I'd begun to wonder if she was trying to goad me into doing it to her. That was out of the question, because I was her friend for one thing, but mainly because her boyfriend really did think I was a pervert. That didn't stop him spanking Katie, and I rather think it was what put the idea into his head, either that or she was tormenting him the same way she used to torment me and he just snapped.

Whatever his reason, I can hardly blame him. Katie was small and pretty, compact rather than petite, but with a chubby, puppy fat bottom it would have been a delight to spank. She also used to go on the beach in bikinis that looked as if she'd borrowed them from a much younger sister, with her breasts barely covered and a serious case of cameltoe, the front pulled tight between the lips of her sex. More of her bottom would be out than in, with her cheeks bulging out to either side and just a hint of the valley between them showing over the top. She used to bounce as she walked, and I remember watching her from the top of a low cliff on one occasion, spellbound by her rear view and wondering how so much flesh could be so perfectly buoyant and why her bikini bottoms didn't give up the unequal struggle and just let it all spill out. I wish they had, because I never saw her bare.

Not surprisingly she turned men's heads, and she knew it. The boyfriend did not approve, and that was the reason he gave for first threatening to spank her unless she went and changed into something more decent, and then picking her up bodily under one arm and applying a half a dozen hard smacks to her wriggling bottom before dropping her on the sand. I was in the beach car park at the time, a couple of hundred yards away, and missed the spectacle, but it's not hard to imagine it, with her tawny blonde curls bouncing to the same rhythm as her smacked bottom and her legs kicking up and down in her shame and frustration as she was held helpless and given what she so thoroughly deserved in front of maybe a couple of hundred people. It's only a shame he didn't complete the job and pull down her bikini pants to give them all a proper show.

Poor Katie wasn't given any choice in the matter, and I wouldn't have included this one but for her reaction and what I learned several years later. At the time I'd assumed that she was an exhibitionist and a tease, but what really turned Katie on was her own embarrassment. When she came to me to show me her bum it wasn't to torment me, or for sympathy, it was because showing her pinked-up cheeks to a known spanking pervert put the final touch to her already raging feelings of erotic humiliation. I didn't know at the time, and nor did her boyfriend, although he got the benefit of it later when they made up with sex in the dunes at the back of the beach. It was only years later when a more mature but far from sober Katie explained her feelings that I learned the truth. She didn't actually like being spanked at all, as such, but from the moment she'd heard that I liked to do it to girls she'd been determined to get it, because it was the most embarrassing thing she could imagine.

Birthday Spanking – Robyn Baker

Robyn Baker was first spanked by a group of her friends. It was a playful punishment on her twenty-first birthday, just a prank and not even overtly sexual, but it was done knickers down and the effect it had on her was considerable, and lasting. This was long before I met her, and the party was a girls-only get together anyway, but it's impossible not to feel a trace of regret for not having been there to witness the event, or preferably to join in with the spanking.

By the time I met Robyn she was in her thirties and married to a friend of mine. He spanks her regularly, as part of foreplay, but it's very much her thing rather than his. Not that he minds, but for her a hot bottom is an essential prerequisite to sex and has been ever since that first spanking. Unfortunately I don't know the full details, only that it happened at the end of a long, drunken night spent with a group of her friends and that the instigator of the spanking was an American. Maybe the idea was in Robyn's head beforehand, because apparently she accepted the idea of a birthday spanking without too much fuss and knelt in an armchair with her bottom stuck out to take it. She is petite, with a small, firm bottom, perhaps rather smaller and firmer then than now, and must have looked a treat with it presented for punishment. I suspect that she was in nothing but a top and panties at the time.

They smacked her with a kitchen spoon, but it hurt too much and she told them to use their hands instead. The American girl – whom I wish I knew because she sounds a lot of fun – then said that if Robyn couldn't take the spoon she'd have to get it bare. This seemed fair to the other girls, who took a good grip on Robyn to keep her in place, pulled down her panties and spanked her bare bottom, each one giving her considerably more than the agreed twenty-one smacks.

Finally they let her go, and she was laughing and swearing she'd get her revenge as she covered herself up, but her bottom was hot in her panties, a sensation she'd never experienced before and which brought the heat to her sex so strongly that she ended up going to the loo to masturbate. I don't know whether she fantasised over what had happened, and I have no reason to believe she is bisexual, so it may be that her reaction was purely physical. That would be unusual, as what's going on in your head is usually crucial to enjoying a spanking, but apparently when her husband does it to her it is purely a physical thing, with nothing to do with submission or humiliation.

Spanked on her Wedding Day – Katie Fletcher

Katie was a girl I first met on holiday many years ago, and

while she and I have never shared more than a kiss, and I haven't seen her in years, we do still have mutual friends, which is how I managed to discover that she was spanked on her wedding night and that it was her first time but not her last. Beyond that I have very few details, but it's easy to picture the scene. Katie is tiny, barely five feet tall, with an elfin figure and melting blue eyes. When I knew her she had her naturally blonde hair cut short with a fringe, giving her a boyish, gamine look that only such a delicate woman could have carried off. I never saw her bare, but her bottom was among the smallest and pertest I've ever seen. She used to wear a blue, one-piece swimming costume that showed her off to perfection, small enough and tight enough to leave plenty of cheek spilling out to either side, and she was also a vision in tight blue jeans. She got her comeuppance about three years after the last time I saw her, so there's no reason to think she had changed very much. I also know she had a white wedding and that the spanking took place in the hotel where the reception was held.

She was always fun, and very playful, so it's easy to imagine her teasing her new husband until he threatened to spank her and then daring him to do it, either in the sure knowledge that she'd get what she was after or prepared to accept the consequences if he had the guts to go through with his threat. Either way she'd have put up a fight, both to preserve some pride and to make him earn his pleasure. In fact she'd probably have been wriggling like anything, even once he'd got her pushed down over the bed, but laughing too, and she did get it, so her beautiful white dress must have been turned up to expose that sweet little bottom, probably covered by white silk panties, or maybe something lacy, although knowing her she might well have gone bare under her wedding dress just for the sake of being cheeky. If she did have panties they certainly came down. After all, why leave her covered?

If they did she must have been quite a sight, her dress and

181

petticoats up high like a huge white flower, framing her little pink bottom and her slender, stocking-clad legs kicking in her panties, her thighs a little open to show off sex lips, either shaved smooth or decorated with a puff of golden fur, and right at the centre her tiny, puckered anus winking in apprehension for what was about to happen to her. I don't suppose it was a very hard spanking, but hopefully she was at least left rosy and warm. It was certainly effective though, because the friend she confessed to, and who subsequently told me, says that Katie was still enjoying regular spankings ten years down the line.

Your Contributions – accounts sent in by spanked girls

SADLY I HAVEN'T MET every girl who's ever been spanked. I already spend far too much time on my obsession, so I suppose it's just as well, but it's nice to know that thanks to the internet the supply is effectively infinite. Almost everybody I spoke to while writing this book knew other people who are into spanking, often in real life, but just as often online. Because a girl's first spanking is nearly always special there were plenty of stories about. Some got passed back to me, some I managed to chase up, and while there were far too many to include every one and most of them were relatively mundane, a few stood out, and those I've included in this section.

Kettle Drum Bum – Christine Hatton

This one is short but sweet, charming and delightfully experimental. It came in late, through an internet forum, and brief though it is I enjoyed Christine's shy enthusiasm so much that I decided to put it in. Christine –

> "Hello. My first spanking was last July, when I asked my boyfriend of two years in a letter. I'd always wanted him to spank me but I'd never had the courage to ask, so I wrote it down, pretty much – 'will you put me over your knee and spank me please' – along with printed off general 'how to' guidelines. He

responded positively, by text – 'a spanking good idea' – and innuendo when chatting online.

When we next met up two weeks later, we happened to be going to a hotel, I acted coy, girly, hopeful. We were relaxing on the bed. I was wearing a white silky underskirt only. I reminded him – was he going to spank me? He said – 'Oh yes, I will, I am'.

He hadn't a clue what to do, so I willingly went over his lap on the bed. He pulled up my underskirt and started to spank, but he was over enthusiastic, often using both hands at once, like he was playing the kettle drums on my bottom, and aiming much too high, at the top of my bottom cheeks, not much at all on my sit spots. They were hard smacks, but as soon as my skin started turning pink the colour stopped him. I felt very pleased that he had done it, and calm, and we cuddled together afterwards. Oh, and I had a sore bottom for the next thirty-six hours."

Self Spanking – Miss Rosy

I couldn't resist this one. Many people would say it doesn't even count, but I found it too charming to ignore. Where it came from, I have no idea. It arrived in an email signed as Miss Rosy but otherwise anonymous, so that's how it's going in, and only slightly tidied up. Miss Rosy -

"I ought to be spanked. I know I ought to be spanked, but who's going to spank me? It's not going to be any man I know. None of them have earned that privilege. Not one of them. The man who spanks me has to be strong. He has to be in control. He has to be completely in control and he has to be a gentleman. I've never met that man and while a lot of men might think they are that man, they're not. That's

184

why I've never been spanked by a man. But I ought to be.

"I ought to be taken down to the shed at the bottom of the garden for a long, hard, old-fashioned spanking. I should have my skirt turned up and my panties pulled down. I should be spanked hard, until I cry, and I should be spanked often, at least once a week. When I've been spanked I should be sent into the corner to stand with my face pressed to the wall and my spanked bottom bare. I'd have to balance a piece of wood from among the chopped logs on my head and if it fell off I'd have to go back for another spanking. That's not going to happen, but it ought to. That's why I spank myself.

"I do it in the woods near my home. It's quiet there and I know I'm not going to get caught. I go right in deep, where it's very lonely and I know nobody can hear. I have a favourite place in among some holly bushes where it's always very pretty and nobody could ever see. I turn up my skirt first. I always wear a skirt for my spankings. Up it comes, just at the back, so my panties show. I stay like that for ages. It feels nice, just knowing my panties show and what I am going to do. After a bit I pull down my panties, not all the way down, but just as far as my man would take them down to get me ready for spanking. I wait again, a long time, just enjoying having my bottom bare in the middle of the woods. I hold off on purpose, to make it feel nicer.

"Then I start to spank. I do it with my fingers first. I do it gently, even though when I think of being spanked in the shed it's always really hard right from the start. That doesn't work when I spank myself. I take it slowly, until my bottom's all lovely and warm and I can feel the heat on my skin. The more I spank and the hotter I get the more daring I get. I'm usually shy and don't show off much, but when I'm spanking myself and I'm warm it feels lovely to stick my bottom right out. I imagine what my man could see while he spanked me and how badly I need that. Sometimes I go down on all fours and imagine being held like that for my spanking.

"When I'm really hot, sometimes I strip right off, but always I stand with my bare bottom showing to the wood and a piece of wood balanced on my head. I play the game, giving myself extra spanks if the wood falls off. Sometimes I'm there for hours, spanking myself and touching myself. Sometimes I have all my clothes off by the end and those are always the best. When I touch myself I think of my man spanking me in the shed. Or sometimes I think I've been caught in the woods and spanked for my bad behaviour. That doesn't make any sense, does it, being spanked for spanking myself? I do wish somebody would do it, but only my man."

The Spanking Machine – Natalia Moreau

This story was sent in from France, by a girl who had heard I was after stories of first spankings from the same friend who introduced me to Emily Evans. I've had to make a few changes to make it suitable for publication, but have done my best to preserve her idiosyncratic style of writing. She assures me it's true, and it is too good a story to be left out in any case. Nor do I have much idea what Natalia looks like, except that she is petite, dark-haired and has what she describes as an "English girl's bottom", which I take to mean plumper than a French girl's bottom. Natalia –

"My first spanking was from Thierry. We would visit

him and he would always make us laugh. He used to make things, with metal, extraordinary things. One time it was a machine to count hen's eggs and let him know in the house when one was laid. Another time it was a lift. You could sit and peddle and go up to a platform in a tree. One time I visited him and he said to me he had something special to show me, a new machine. He took me out to his shed, where he made everything, and there was a strange machine, like a bicycle. More like an exercise bicycle. There was no front wheel and no seat, but the back wheel was there and stuck onto it was a big leather paddle, like a fly swatter.

"I asked Thierry what it was for. He said it was for giving naughty girls a spanking. I thought he was making a joke and laughed, but he said I should go on it. I wasn't sure, but he said I must. I went on, standing up on the pedals, but he told me to pretend there was a seat. I felt silly, ridiculous, with my bottom stuck out like I was trying to go to the loo. I knew when I started to pedal the big leather paddle would smack me on my bottom. I went very slowly, but it still came up fast and whack! right on my bottom. We both laughed. He said to pedal faster and I said okay, making the paddle smack on my bottom again and again. It was all a joke, just that, except that the smacks were giving my bottom a funny warm feeling.

"He asked if it hurt at all. I said no, it felt quite nice. He said I should turn up my dress, and okay, it was Thierry, so that was good. But, I was on the bicycle, the spanking bicycle, so he turned up my dress, right up, to make my knickers show. I pedalled, and the paddle spanked me on my knickers, but after a few moments my dress fell down. Thierry said I should take off my dress and when I said no he said not to be foolish. I had no bra and I was ashamed to show my chest, but again he said not to be foolish, and he was Thierry. And so, off came my dress.

"Again I went on the spanking bicycle. Now the smacks were on my knickers and it felt hotter than before. Strange too, and nice in a funny way. I was very ashamed because of the way my chest jiggled when I pedalled and the way my bottom showed, because my knickers were getting wet and I was sure he would see and know it wasn't sweat. Again he asked if it hurt at all and again I said no. He said the proper way was to be bare and I should pull down my knickers. I said no but he pulled them down anyway and I didn't stop him. He was excited and me as well, but we pretended it was just to test the machine. Again I pedalled and now the paddle spanked me on my bare bottom. Now it made my flesh sting but I wanted it to and pedalled faster and even faster. He pulled my knickers right down so I knew he could see my cunt and see I was wet. I felt very ashamed, and dirty, so I didn't mind when he took out his cock.

"Thierry began to wank. He was watching me on the spanking bicycle and wanking. I pedalled faster, showing him, terribly ashamed of myself but also proud because he was so big and excited for me. I thought he would fuck me, but he did it in his hand, but very close, so when he ejaculated it went over my bottom. I could feel his come, wet on my hot skin and I felt extraordinarily dirty. I knew he had put me on the spanking bicycle so he could come, obviously, but I didn't mind. Even when he put a hand between my thighs I didn't mind. He said I needed to come too and he was going to make me. I let him, with my bottom stuck right out and my feet still on the pedals

while he fiddled with my cunt. He touched my
bottom too, feeling my hot flesh and rubbing his own
mess over my skin. He talked to me too, saying I was
a naughty girl to let him take my knickers down. He
said he loved my bottom and he said he wanted to
kiss and lick me to make me better after my spanking
but I was wishing he would shut up and spank me
more while he made me come. I said he could and he
did, using his hand to spank me while he masturbated
my cunt until I got there. It was the best.

"That was my first spanking but not my last!"

Scrumping Spanking – Miss Nightingale

I wasn't at all sure about including this piece. For one thing
it came from an unexpected angle, which I can't go into
except to say that it relates to one of my other contributions,
intimately. It is also very close to the bone, but it is
ultimately consensual and erotic for the receiver, so I let it
through. I also felt that it deserved to be recorded, both for
curiosity's sake and because it apparently dates from the
1930s, making it the oldest contribution to this book by over
twenty years. Miss Nightingale is the name the lady who
wrote to me gave as her maiden name. The original letter
was hand-written, long and extremely insightful but I've had
to cut it down considerably to make it suitable for
publication. Miss Nightingale –

"I would like my experience to be included in your
book. Before I start you need to understand how I
feel about spanking. For me it was simply something
that happened, a part of life. I had no frame of
reference against which to compare my experiences.
There were no books on the subject, certainly not that
I had access too. As for the internet, no such thing

189

had so much as been imagined. Nowadays it is very different. I didn't even feel the guilt that marks ------'s account of her own first spanking. For me, being spanked was part of everyday life. I saw it as the consequence of my behaviour, neither more nor less. If I misbehaved there was a possibility that I would be spanked, as simple as that. That was acceptable and that was what I understood. What I did not understand was my reaction to the thought of being spanked. In this liberated, informed age this may seem difficult to believe, but I didn't even understand the idea of sexual arousal. Nobody had taught me anything, save that I was expected to submit myself to my husband in some intimate but mysterious way. He would know what to do, I was told and I found the thought immensely appealing. I also expected him to spank me and that thought was also immensely appealing, although I could not truly have explained why. I did know that my feelings were connected with the warm, luxurious sensations I enjoyed every time I thought about him spanking me.

"I now know all about endorphins and the way spanking stimulates the genitals, but at the time I'm not sure that the medical profession understood such things, and if they did the information was not about to be made available to a respectable young lady living in rural Devon. All I knew was that the thought of being spanked gave me the most delightful feelings. First there would be pain, alongside the feelings of indignity and contrition that went with having my bottom laid bare, but the pleasure that came with that far outweighed the bad feelings. I came to crave spanking.

"I needed somebody who would spank me, but I had no immediate prospect of marriage and it never occurred to me to ask for a spanking from one of the young men I knew, especially as I didn't consider any of them suitable husband material. It would have been scandalous, especially as having my bottom laid bare was an important part of what for me had become a ritual. I'd have much rather asked one of my friends to spank me and I did consider the notion, only to reject it as impossibly embarrassing. You have to understand that while it was perfectly normal for a young woman to be spanked, the idea of a young woman asking to be spanked was an impossible outrage. I would have to give somebody an excuse to punish me.

"Had I had any sense at all, or patience, I would have waited until I was married, and when I eventually did get married I used to be spanked regularly, usually on a Sunday after church. At the time that was still over a year away and I had no idea what the future would bring. Instead I took to trespassing on Mr S-----'s land, a shortcut between my house and the village. Mr S----- was an elderly, mean and above all bad-tempered farmer. Being on his land filled me with apprehension, but also desire, because he'd twice threatened me with spanking when I was a little girl. Sure enough, he caught me, and he threatened me again, but he didn't do it, which left me in a state of frustration I'd never known before but which was to get worse. I was more scared than ever, but I had to go on, and the next time he caught me and threatened to,'give me the hiding I deserved' – I told him he wouldn't dare.

"I thought that would make him do it, and I could see he wanted to, but somehow he held his temper in check. All I could do was try again, but not only did I continue to cross his land but I took to scrumping apples from his orchard. The next time he caught me I had my dress held up to carry a dozen or more of his best apples, only things hadn't quite gone to plan. He wasn't alone. His son was with him, a big, strapping lad a couple of years younger than me whose invitation to a local dance I'd turned down only the week before.

"Maybe it was because his son was there and he couldn't be seen to back down. Maybe he'd just had enough of my behaviour, but this time he didn't even threaten. He just told me what was going to happen, that I was going to get a spanking, then and there. I froze, unable to move or resist him in any way, although I was complaining bitterly about my treatment as he grabbed me and bundled me across his knee. My dress was already half up because of the way I'd been carrying the apples, which were now all over the ground, and as he caught hold of the hem I remember how extraordinarily strong my feelings were. The idea of having my bottom laid bare, and in front of Lias, who was standing there gaping like a goldfish, was absolutely unbearable and at one and the same time perfectly desirable. I'd never felt such deep shame, nor such excitement.

"Not that it made the slightest difference what I felt. My dress came up and my drawers were pulled open with two swift motions and there I was, the way I'd imagined myself so often, laid bare-bottomed over a man's knee and about to be spanked. I couldn't imagine how I could possibly have been stupid enough to let myself get into that situation, especially when he began to spank me, because it hurt like anything, but at the same time I was in heaven. Just knowing he had my bottom bare made me feel faint and the pain of the spanking robbed me of whatever resistance I might have had left. He spanked me long and hard, but the worst of it, and the best, was being bare in front of Lias, whom I'd rejected. He was obviously enjoying the view as well, and after he'd seen me like that, what was I to do? We were married less than a year later, the following June."

Hand and Hairbrush – Cara Marie

With this entry we go from the earliest spanking in the book to the most recent. As you'll see, it shows just how much easier it is to get what you want these days than it used to be!

Cara Marie is a very beautiful Italian-American girl newly introduced to the US spanking scene. She met a friend of mine who was on a spanking tour of the States. I contacted her to ask for her story, and here it is. Cara Marie–

"When I was in college, I lived in the same house with seven other girls during my senior year. Can you believe that? We actually managed to squeeze eight girls into one house. Well, eight girls plus one girl's fiancé. Jon practically lived with us from the day we moved into the house. We doubted that he had an apartment of his own because he was always at ours with Lexi.

"One evening, right before we would all go away for the winter holidays, all eight of us girls were sitting around watching *America's Next Top Model*. The show wasn't really my cup of tea, but the other seven girls would cancel all of their plans to see it, and it was rare to get all eight of us in the same place at one time. So I decided, tonight would be the night to sit through *America's Next Top Model* with my eight roommates and Jon.

"Lexi that evening was being quite a brat. Jon had gone to the store and picked up munchies and soda for the get-together. Now, he was busy in the kitchen putting everything into bowls and on platters. He asked Lexi for help, and he was greeted with a prompt, 'Fuck you!'. The rest of us snapped our heads around. None of us had ever heard Lexi talk that way. She rarely raised her voice, and swear words never escaped her lips. About a minute passed, and no one said anything. Jon came coolly around the corner and said, 'Lexi, I'm tired and frustrated with how you've been treating me all day today. I am not a housewife, I do not need to clean up after you, and you can help while I'm getting ready for your party. This attitude has to stop'. Without another word, he grabbed her wrist, stood her up from the couch, and took her upstairs. Downstairs, the other girls and I exchanged puzzled glances. What was going on?

"A few minutes later, we heard something that sounded like nails being hammered into the wall, followed by Lexi screaming. I quickly realized she was getting a spanking. I was giggling. Some of the other girls were giggling too. A couple of them had horrified looks on their faces. I went downstairs to my room. I could still hear the spanking going on two floors above and I was increasingly aware that I was getting wet. With the spanking still going on upstairs and with Lexi now crying hysterically, I sat down to my computer, and googled – 'Erotic spanking.' After looking at a few links, I found Shadow Lane.

"It wasn't until later that I found out Jon and Lexi were in a domestic discipline relationship, and I do wonder if they didn't set their show up on purpose, for kicks. That's what got me into it anyhow. After joining Shadow Lane I quickly started to get offers. I met a man named John (not the same Jon as Lexi's fiancé) at the metro in Washington, DC. He was going to be my first spanker, and I was so nervous. I started to go up the stairs to exit the subway at least three times. I kept going back down, getting cold feet, and wanting to get back on the metro and go home. But I didn't. I got up my courage, went up the stairs and found John outside. He was a big, tall guy – easily twice my size and my weight, but he wasn't intimidating. He really looked like a big teddy bear. I instantly felt safe, and thought it was OK to have dinner with him.

"We went out to an Italian restaurant, and we talked about limits, and safe words, and what I wanted out of my first spanking. I made up a reason that I needed to be disciplined for. I told John that I was falling behind on my school work and that I had a case of "senior-itis." It totally wasn't true – I was 100% on top of my school work and was looking at potentially being a valedictorian. I guess I just thought I needed to be spanked for something!

"After dinner, we went back to his apartment, and he took me by the hand into the living room. He asked me if I knew why I was getting a spanking. All I could do was nod. I was so nervous that if I started speaking I wasn't sure anything would come out. So I nodded, and he nodded back. He stood me up, took down my jeans and guided me over his lap. Once over his lap, he pulled down my panties. I knew that would happen, because we had talked about it, but I was surprised when it happened. My hand instinctively went back, but by the time it got there, my bottom was already bare. He grabbed my wrist and pinned it against my back. I wasn't going anywhere.

"He started spanking me, and after a few swats, it was already starting to hurt. I was never spanked as a child, so it was a completely new experience to me. After about a minute, I thought my bottom was one fire. Every swat seemed exponentially harder than the last one! I didn't cry, but I was getting wetter and wetter as the spanking went on, and when I wasn't concentrating on the pain in my bottom, I was praying that John didn't notice that I was dripping.

"After what seemed like an eternity, he stopped. I thought he was done, and I went to get up, but he pushed me back down. 'Not yet,' he said, 'I'm not done with you yet.' He picked up a hairbrush that was lying on the coffee table next to the couch. I couldn't believe I had missed its presence! The first smack of the hairbrush sent me screaming. It wasn't that hard a smack, but it stung like a million little bees. John only gave me ten swats with the hairbrush, but it seemed to take for ever. Time stood still. I started crying, more from the emotional release of being over someone's knee for the first time than from the pain of the spanking. When it was done, he held me in his arms, let me cry it out, and when I had calmed down he flipped me over on my tummy and rubbed some lotion on my bottom. He kept the lotion in the freezer, so it was icy cold, and felt amazing on my hot bottom."

More Contributions – accounts from other spankers

WHEN I FIRST SET out to write this book I had intended to use a mixture of my own reminiscences and interviews with girls who like to be spanked. However, girls who like to be spanked usually have partners who like to do the spanking, while so many of the girls also enjoy spanking each other that to find one who doesn't is rare. Because of that I soon had some wonderful first spanking stories coming in at second-hand, stories far too good not to be included.

Being a Beast – from Phil Kemp

Phil has been a devoted spanker since before I was born and is no less keen now, after more than five decades of applying his hand to squirming female bottom cheeks at every opportunity. He is also a writer, specialising in short stories, and author of *Blushing at Both Ends*, a highly successful collection, some of it drawn from real life. He has given plenty of girls their first spanking, but chose to tell me about what was also the first he ever gave and which makes a very sweet story. Phil –

> "I'm pleased to say that the first spanking I ever gave was also her first, and it was a proper, bare-bottom, over the knee spanking, not just a few pats on the seat of a girl's jeans. She was my cousin. That's acceptable is it, for the book?"

197

"Don't worry. I spanked my cousin too, and she's going in. I expect it happens quite a lot."

"You're probably right, for sex anyway. After all, we all need somebody to experiment with. Mine was called Jenny, and she was the youngest of three girls, much the prettiest too. I used to go there every summer, to my uncle's place in the country. Jenny was a couple of years younger than me; been playmates since we were children, but as she matured I couldn't help but notice what a lovely, spankable little bottom she had."

"So you were keen to do it from the first?"

"Very keen. I've always liked spanking. After all, it's what girls' bottoms are for."

"I can go along with that, a design classic I'd say."

"Exactly, why else would they be so well padded? Jenny certainly was, slim but with the plumpest little bottom you can possibly imagine, and perfectly rounded. I might not have dared to spank her though, had it not been for what happened one morning at breakfast. Her sisters were quite a bit older than her, and still used to treat her as a child, especially Monica, the eldest. Jenny was being difficult, first saying she wanted eggs and then changing her mind when the pan was already boiling and pinching a piece of Monica's toast. She was grinning at me as she spread butter and honey on it, and I shared the joke, grinning back, until Monica turned around. She was not happy about it, and told Jenny flatly to grow up before turning back to the cooker. Jenny immediately pinched the second piece of toast, but Monica had been expecting that and turned back immediately. She was genuinely cross, and she shouted at Jenny, calling her a little brat, but when Jenny answered her back she said something I'll never forget if I live to be a

198

hundred – 'If you're going to behave like a child, then I'll treat you like a child. Come here'. Jenny knew exactly what Monica meant, and she let out a squeal like a steam train as she realised she was going to be spanked, and in front of me. She let Monica do it though, really quite meek as she went over her sister's knee for twenty swats on the seat of her pyjamas. Maybe she knew she'd get it anyway and didn't want to make an exhibition of herself, or maybe she thought that if she put up a fight she might get her pyjama trousers pulled down, I don't know, but she took it, about twenty hard swats. Her face was bright red afterwards, and I was imagining her bum the same colour. But the thing was, the moment Monica's back was turned Jenny was grinning at me again, deeply embarrassed, but still grinning. "

"Maybe she goaded Monica into spanking her on purpose?"

"Looking back, she probably did. At the time I was just grateful that I had a napkin to conceal my raging erection. Not surprisingly I couldn't stop thinking about what had happened, and just to watch the way Jenny's bottom moved under her jeans made my fingers itch with the desire to give her the same treatment her sister had."

"I know exactly how you felt."

"I still didn't dare, although we were together most of the time. A couple of days after the spanking we went up to the attic, to fetch something, I think, but we ended up rummaging around. I found a box full of the old penny dreadful novels and started to read one. Jenny got bored and sneaked up behind me with a moth-eaten old feather boa and rubbed it in my face. I wasn't expecting it at all, and I got a mouthful of mouldy old feathers and dust and cobwebs. She was laughing at me, and I must have looked a sight, but she seemed to be nervous too, with one hand half over her mouth as if she was scared of my reaction. Suddenly I had my excuse. I had to do it, if it was the last thing I did, so I grabbed her and sat down on the box, hauling her across my knee. She knew exactly what was going to happen and was struggling like anything and threatening me, but she couldn't stop giggling either so I didn't let up. I was determined to get her jeans down too, because I'd thought about doing it so often and because otherwise it wouldn't have seemed like a proper spanking, and she fought like anything to stop me getting at the button under her tummy. I wouldn't have had the guts to take her knickers down, but her jeans were so tight they came down anyway, and all of a sudden I had her sweet little bottom bare in front of me. It was the first time I'd had a girl's bum nude, let alone nude over my lap and ready for spanking. She was still giggling too, and obviously didn't mind having her jeans and knickers down in front of me all that much, so I began to spank. I still remember how her bum felt, soft and firm all at the same time, and the way her cheeks bounced as I smacked them, and kept parting to show a little puff of hair between. I was in heaven."

"I can imagine."

"I wanted to spank her properly, the way her sister had done, but as I started to make the smacks harder she began to protest, calling me a beast and wriggling about on my lap. I didn't stop, because I rather liked being called a beast and her wriggling was making the show she was giving of her bare bum even ruder. Besides, I still hadn't managed to get all the muck out of my mouth and I felt she deserved what she was getting. So I carried on until her bottom was a lovely shade of warm red, and by then I'd realised that this was something I wanted to do … no, something I had to do. I'd always wanted to do it. When she started to cry I finally took pity on her and let her up. She was still calling me a beast, as she stood there rubbing her bottom and trying to inspect her cheeks by the dim light from the attic windows, but she didn't bother to pull up her jeans and knickers, despite being bare right in front of me. Maybe it was just that I'd seen it all anyway, because girls are often like that, but although she kept calling me a beast she definitely had mixed feelings about her spanking. Over the next few weeks she was constantly goading me, angling for more spankings, which she got, several times, and at the very end of my stay she admitted she liked it and said something really sweet, that she liked to be spanked by me instead of her sisters, because they only did it when they were angry, but I did it because I liked her."

That was the end of Phil's official interview, but we continued to talk for over an hour, swapping spanking reminiscences from across the years. It's a rare privilege for me to be able to talk to somebody whose experience goes back before my own, a full twenty years in this case, and I always enjoy hearing about spankings administered before my time. His best stories included a beautiful and very bossy German girl who goaded him into spanking her as she sunbathed, with her bikini pants pulled down at the back to bare her bottom. She remained firmly in charge, telling him what to do even as she began to stick up her rapidly reddening bottom in excitement and finally dismissing him when she was hot enough. He was left to watch as she slipped a hand down under her tummy to find her sex and brought herself to orgasm with her well smacked cheeks thrust high, her bottom hole, pussy and busy fingers on full show.

Then there was a trip to Mykonos in his late teens. Phil spanked another German girl during an idyllic day nude sunbathing on a deserted beach. Later, when the girl's travelling companion found out about it, she demanded rather indignantly why Phil hadn't spanked her too. As she was just as pretty as her friend, he was glad to oblige. A little later, at university, one of Phil's friends was dumped rather heartlessly by his girlfriend. The next time Phil met her he berated her for her cruelty, to which she responded with the classic line, "Well, what are you going to do about it – spank me?" He took her back to his rooms in college and did just that. Since she knew Phil was into spanking, it's more than likely that's what she was angling for, and that illustrates an important point. If you want plenty of girls to spank, make sure they know you're a spanker.

Secret Spanking – from Madame Caramel

The majority of girls who like to be spanked enjoy or even prefer other women dishing it out, and although most have their first experience with a man I found plenty of exceptions. One came from the magnificent Madame Caramel, professional domina and organiser of Club Black Whip, who provided me with a delightful story of a fellow dominant woman who came to her for a first, and very secret, spanking.

Caramel's own background is fascinating. Brought up among the political elite of Angola, she hah been used to automatic respect from everybody around her and maids to answer her every whim. Even if she wanted a glass of milk there would be somebody to fetch it for her. All that came to an end when she left the country, first for Portugal and then for Britain, but she still feels that it is natural for her to be served. With that goes forceful, innate dominance, intelligence, charm, extraordinarily good humour, a pretty face and a chest capable of making an Egyptian mummy sit up and pay attention. I was also struck by her confidence. Many dominant women feel the need to assert themselves when with their male counterparts, but Caramel was entirely at ease from the moment we met.

She was watching Angola play Malawi at football in the African Nations Cup, with great excitement, but only at the end of the match did she trouble to point out her uncle among the men in the Presidential box. By then she had made me coffee and brought out a plate of spiced sausages, shown me around her house, passed a knowledgeable comment on the bottle of Mercurey I'd brought and corrected my pronunciation of the vineyards around Lisbon. What she hadn't done was tell me anything at all about the first-time spanking she'd dished out to her friend, but we got there eventually. Caramel –

"You're going to have to change a lot of details, because this is secret, but when I met her I was the house domme at a club in ... let's say Blackpool, and we'll call her Scarlett, although I'd better not say why. She's very beautiful, small and just so, with very pale skin and a delicate face, tattoos and piercings too, so a really strong fetish style. I was dominating a man, a bit of CBT ..."

"Which is, for the readers?"

"Cock and ball torture. She asked if she could join in, and if I'd show her how to handle him properly. We had a lot of fun, with him, and with her boyfriend, so when we were done I gave her my card. That was it, and I didn't hear from her for months, until she emailed me out of the blue, and after passing messages back and forth for a while she confessed to a submissive streak and asked if I would help her explore it in private, without anybody else knowing, especially her boyfriend. My reply was yes, and I'd do it for free."

"Were you just being generous, or did you have another reason?"

"I liked her, and I wanted it to be special. It's never quite the same if money is changing hands."

"Obviously she accepted?"

"Like a shot. We arranged everything and she came down to see me a couple of weeks later. She was nervous, so I took her for cocktails first to help her relax, then back home and up to my playroom, which you've seen."

"Yes. I love the way it looks fairly innocent, a little sultry perhaps but no more than that, until you open the wardrobe with all the gear inside."

"My throne might be a bit of a giveaway too."

"Only if you're in the know."

"She was. I sat down on it and she immediately got on her knees in front of me and started to explain about how she had wanted to submit to me from the moment we met and how often she'd fantasised about the moment. She said she wanted to worship me, and that I could do whatever I pleased. I began by undressing her. She was in jeans and a blouse, with heels, but all very ordinary, but underneath she had on brand new knickers and bra, all pink and lacy, very different to the hard, gothic person she'd been at the club. I took everything off, to leave her completely naked, and ordered her to climb on to my bed and pose for me, showing off her lovely pale body in all sorts of positions. She was very nervous, but she was obedient too, and did as she was told, even when it meant exposing herself completely. When I told her to caress her body she hesitated, but only for a moment. I had stayed on my throne all this time, since I'd got her undressed, just watching, but once I could see that she was warming up I went to her and took over, first caressing her body in turn, before making her lie face down on the bed. I began to spank her bottom, very gently at first, then gradually harder. She'd began to sigh at first, then started moaning and panting, pushing her bum up to the smacks as her cheeks grew redder. My hand had begun to sting, which I like, but she had given in to me completely and obviously needed more. I switched to a paddle, using it hard, until her bum was blazing red and she was wriggling and moaning. She was mine completely, because I'd punished her, I'm sure you know how that is? I took baby oil and began to rub it in, caressing her hot cheeks, and in between. Spanking makes me horny, but this was something else, and she was worse, desperate to worship me with her tongue. I still made her go slow, smelling my skin and tasting me before I allowed her to get down on her knees again and lick me to orgasm while she played with herself."

"Wonderful, thanks. That's among the most sensual spankings I've heard about. She was very lucky she came to you for her first time."

"I think so, and we've been friends ever since."

"That's not surprising, with you. Sometimes it would be, but with you I can see that she could submit to you completely when you play together but otherwise be perfectly good friends."

A Naughty Nurse – from Mark Langton

I met Mark when he and I sat together on a panel of judges. It was a talent show, after a fashion, with couples coming up on stage to show off their skills with the Scots tawse, girls and boys both, each bottom displayed to the judges and crowd before being expertly smacked. The tawse is a notoriously tricky implement to use. Thick, flexible leather does wonders for a recalcitrant bottom, but it needs to be guided on to its target, not easy at the best of times, and especially hard to deliver with both accuracy and force. I was impressed by Mark's knowledge of the subject and after the competition we talked for a while, on spankings we'd given and girls we'd known who like to be spanked. He'd given plenty of initiations in his time, and so I asked him for an interview. Sadly that proved impractical, but he did send a contribution, which I include here precisely as it came in. Mark –

"She was a ward sister in a London hospital. Judith. Pretty, with a cheerful heart-shaped face, hazel eyes and dark wavy hair. Vivacious and smiled a lot. But I didn't really notice her – as a woman – until the pair of us were asked to give some evening training sessions for nurses in Enfield. I was living in the East End and drove us up there. Two hours in a chilly lecture room, every Tuesday for six weeks.

"On the way back, down Green Lanes, we were hungry and stopped at a Turkish café for saveloys and chips. It was fun. He face shone when she was animated and I was becoming aware of the firm body under the suit she was wearing. Back in the car she gave me a kiss on the cheek. 'Thanks, that was lovely.'

"We parted with a slightly less chaste kiss when I dropped her outside the block in Whitechapel where sisters had their hospital flats. Sorry to disappoint you, no shagging that night. But by the end of week two we had gone out together and found we enjoyed each other's company. In week three, we went back to my flat, down by the canal, and became lovers. Judith was twenty-six and coy about previous men. There had been some, because she certainly knew what she wanted and what to give. She could make love fiercely and wildly, but also generously and tenderly. She often fell asleep with her head on my chest or tucked under my arm. She was delightful to wake up to. And she could dress in seconds when called to an emergency, pulling up knickers and tights in one amazing continuous movement, slipping into the blue dress and popping on the ridiculously complex white cap that went back to Nurse Cavell's time. Add her dark blue, scarlet-lined cape and she looked angelic. And she'd been screwing like a tigress only five minutes before.

"We were both very tied to the hospital, where I was a junior doctor, but there was time for trips to riverside pubs like the Prospect of Whitby, going to the theatre, out for meals in the Indian restaurants all around us. Looking at the Thames from a balcony at the Prospect one evening, my arm round her, she put down her drink and turned to look at me. 'You know, I think I'm falling in love with you, Mark. I love being in charge on the ward, I'm not a wimp and I know I can be bossy, but you make me feel so comfortable – and safe.'

I gave her a big hug. 'Hmm. Perhaps you need a man to take you in hand, young Judith, someone even bossier than you?' I patted her on the bottom. She wriggled sexily and giggled. 'Maybe I do – a strong man who's also very gentle. You know, I sometimes think maybe I've found one?'

"Within a month we were seen by our friends as an item. We spent our spare time together. We made love a lot, usually in an equal partnership, both being inventive, both sometimes taking a lead. But other times I could tell she just wanted to be taken like a whore – kneeling naked on the bed, head in the pillows, sticking her bum up and wriggling lewdly to be screwed hard from behind as I gripped her hips and thrust voraciously, almost roughly, until we came together.

"But I still hadn't mentioned it. My dread secret. I could never explain why – I can't to this day – but, deep within my psyche, a part of my sexuality was – and is – aroused strongly by the exquisite curves of female bottoms, by spanking, by role playing in which my partner is willing to go across my knee, to be given a spanking that is real and stings but gives her pleasure. I'm at the soft end of the spectrum – no blood – but cuffs and straps, martinets, canes and all the rest are also part of it. I had played these emotionally overpowering games with a few like-minded friends I had found, but never with a feisty woman like Judith with whom I was – well – falling in love. Never with a girl I was serious about. Who I could see making a life with me, building a family? Growing old together? Well, all that was a long way down the line. Maybe it would never happen. But I sensed we were both rather hoping it might. So how the hell was I to tell her? Tell her an important part of me, an essential part of me was, well, perverted. It could blow the whole thing.

"Curiously it was a friend of Judith's who helped to solve the problem. Lalage was beautiful in a pre-Raphaelite sort of way. She was a teacher in a primary school not far away. Her accent was cut glass, she came from a grand old catholic family, lived in a nice flat in Chelsea and travelled on the District Line every day to teach the great unwashed. Her superiority got right up my nose.

"We were in the Blind Beggar pub, where the Krays

had ruled their criminal empire, the three of us drinking pints early in the evening. Lalage was talking about the school, a catholic one of course, how the children thrived under a degree of discipline. This was forty years ago and most schools still had corporal punishment. That's what we were discussing. Lalage was matter-of-fact, Judith oddly tense and asking questions. Did girls get punished as well as boys? Was it on the bare?

"They did, and it was across their knickers. Conversation moved on, but later, as we walked back to my flat, thoughtfully, hand in hand, it began again. She had never been spanked, but after a while she said something wonderful – 'Maybe – maybe – it might just be right for bossy grown-up women?'

"She was talking about spanking. But was she responding to something she'd sensed in me, or was she responding to something that lurked in her? I put my arms round her and gave her a lingering kiss. 'There's only one way to find out.'

Back in the flat, I drew the curtains and we both had a glass of wine, Judith looking uncertain and nervous. I stood up and so did she, putting her arms slowly round my neck (she was six inches shorter) and giving me a tentative kiss. 'Oh, Mark, I'm not sure. I'm afraid it will hurt too much – and I'm afraid my bum will look ridiculous. I'll feel stupid.' But she wasn't saying no. 'Promise you won't laugh.' 'Not unless you do.'

"She stood there shifting nervously from foot to foot. 'Then do it, darling – and do it now, before I get really terrified and change my mind!' She paused uncertainly – 'I haven't been … been spanked before. How – how do you want me?'

"I put my hands one on each of her shoulders and

met her eyes firmly. She looked back with a sudden mischievous sparkle. 'Take off your dress, Judith.' She responded obediently, slipping it daintily to the floor. I helped her to take off her bra to reveal those beautiful firm breasts, her nipples already hard. Then her shoes and tights. I sat down and she stood before me in a golden light from the single lamp on the table. Her face was apprehensive again as she bit her lip. Shoulders quite broad, flat tummy, neatly trimmed dark triangle above those strong nurse's legs. 'You look so beautiful.'

"She smiled hesitantly, but I responded sternly. 'Bend over my knee.' I put out my hands to help as she draped herself across my lap, balancing on hands spread on the carpet. I landed two sharp smacks on the seat of her tiny black knickers and she gasped. Then I took the waistband. She stiffened – 'Oh, no,' – but raised her hips as I rolled them slowly, very slowly down to her knees.

"Her legs, broad thighs with a hint of strong muscle, tapering to slim calves, stretched out to toes digging into the carpet. I started to stroke her bottom, luxuriating in its flawless beauty. It swelled out sensuously from a narrow waist – two full, fleshy globes, a hint of dark fuzz peeping from the deep, mysterious cleft between them. Judith had a bum that was round but firm. Her skin was almost honey-coloured and felt beautifully soft, like silk or a peach, and I caressed it gently with my right hand while my left held her firmly in place. She sighed and her body relaxed – 'Oh, this bit's lovely. But my bum must look enormous!'

"'You have an absolutely beautiful bottom, my darling.' I started to smack it gently, starting low down on each cheek, where they curved to tuck into the crease at the top of her thighs. There was silence from under her mop of dark hair, but her body wriggled and jerked with each slap. 'It flawless, sexy and the only thing wrong is that it's nowhere near pink enough yet.'

"I started to spank harder, moving my hand all over her bottom, up and down, a few slaps to the side of those reddening cheeks. She was panting now and giving breathless little cries – 'Oh – ouch – ow! It hurts!' Her legs parted, revealing a tuft of dark pubic hair and the tantalising oval of her swelling and opening labia. 'It's meant to hurt, girl, and you jolly well deserve it.' I used my left hand to part the cheeks of her bottom, revealing the inner flesh of that exciting cleft and the puckered little pink star of her anus. With two fingers I spanked her sharply all down the crease, especially over and around that little star. I thought she might be shocked or embarrassed, but she squirmed with what was clearly wild pleasure. 'Oh, yes – oh please – oh Christ!' I returned my left hand firmly to the small of her back and spanked even harder, two resounding ones at the top of each thigh, then a volley from cheek to cheek, and another of real stingers across the middle, over her bumhole.

"By now I knew it was OK. She was wriggling and squirming luxuriantly, bottom bouncing, yelping at each stinging smack. Her legs were scissoring wildly, knickers slipping down to one ankle and flying off. Between her thighs the knot of her sex shone with moisture, the musky scent of arousal hung in the air. Her bottom was turning crimson. "I'm going to give you twelve very hard ones, young lady, six on each side. Are you ready?"

"'Oh, no! Yes, I am, Sir.' Her bum thrust up to meet the first whack as it cracked into her right buttock and

211

she howled louder at each one: 'Aargh – ouch – OW – no more, please!'

"As she winced and writhed at the last of the dozen, I wanted to show how much I loved her and slipped my fingers between her thighs to seek out her clitoris and go deep into her warm, wet, lustful vagina. 'Ooh, oh my God, yes, my darling!' Suddenly her whole body arched upwards, she was crying out and came in a series of uncontrollable, rolling orgasms.

"Afterwards she lay there for a while, spent and naked over my knee, as I stroked her red hot bottom and told her I loved her. When I eased her up, her eyes were shining and wet with tears. She kissed me. 'Thank you. You know, I thought it would hurt and be so embarrassing , but I'd do it just for you. And it did hurt – you really whacked me like a naughty little girl, but it was amazing. I thought I might hate it – I had no idea I'd like it so much.' I dried her eyes. 'Don't look so worried, lover, I'm crying because I'm really happy and my bum's glowing and I feel horny as hell!'

"So did I and we fell into bed together. And the rest of the story? Well, that's for another day, but we did stay together, if you want to know, and went all over the world. Forty years on we live in a Devon farmhouse, just put the grandchildren on the train to London. And I spanked Judith when we got home."

Musical Bottoms – from TV Joanna

I had more than enough material to complete this book by the time I managed to track down the notorious Joanna, but I didn't feel it would be complete without her account. Four of the girls I'd interviewed had taken their first spanking from her, three of them exclusively so, while I'd met several

212

others who'd either been spanked by her or done the spanking. Even in the obsessive world of spanking enthusiasts her dedication was extraordinary.

Once I'd managed to get in touch I found her both friendly and accommodating. The charm that had enabled her to tempt so many girls out of their knickers was evident from the first, and as I travelled down to her South London home my only concern was for my own etiquette. Would he, or she, be his mundane, male self, or her glamorous, female persona?

She was Joanna, over six feet tall in her strappy turquoise and white platform heels, with white fishnet stockings, a turquoise micro-skirt and a lightweight white top accessorised with a white belt and plenty of bling, all topped off with honey-blonde hair. Her manner was courteous, slightly tart, slightly firm, quickly setting me at ease as she ushered me up to her boudoir, where the interview was to be conducted. I've been in a great many dungeons and playrooms, most of which have been decorated in black, perhaps with highlights of red and purple. Joanna's boudoir was rather different, the walls painted a combination of Dulux "Sexy Pink" and lavender, the upholstery for the main part pink but also showing zebra stripe, gold and scarlet. There were also several items of play furniture and a great many CP implements, including whips, canes, paddles and even an old-fashioned carpet beater. I was immediately fascinated and spent a happy few minutes admiring the fixtures and fittings while she made coffee.

With coffee mugs in hand we began to talk, discussing technique and the virtues of different implements, swapping spanking stories and comparing notes on mutual acquaintances, especially those I'd spanked but she had given their first experience. Joanna –

"I love spanking. I love everything about spanking, giving it and taking it, the sensual pleasure of it, the

213

way it makes you want to fuck. Best of all I love introducing girls to spanking."

"You seem to have a knack for that."

"I'd like to think so. I do have a lot of experience, and I do think it's very important that a girl's first experience should be a good one. I know too many girls who've been put off because some guy's just waded in, too hard and too fast."

"I've heard that again and again, but all the girls I've spoken to say you make it very sensual. So just how many girls have you given their first spanking?"

"Thirty-three. That's out of over three hundred I've spanked."

"Three hundred? I've spoken to people who consider themselves lucky to have had a single spanking partner, if that. So how do you manage it, and when did you start?"

"Not all that long ago, maybe fifteen years. I used to work in fetish clubs, setting up mainly, so I was always about and got to know people and would play a lot. Often people would watch and then ask me to spank them in turn."

"Including Emily Evans?"

"Emily Evans? Oh, Emily. Yes, she was number … twenty-eight."

"With her boyfriend's full encouragement, so she tells me?"

"Yes. I'm always very careful not to cut partners out, but I think it's something to do with me being TV as well. They don't see Joanna as a threat. I have a reputation too. People know that I like to make a girl's first experience really special so they recommend me to new girls. Usually they come back for more. Just about always in fact. The knack is to start slow and easy, not too hard, with plenty of talking to soothe her feelings. I start by using a particular rhythm to warm her cheeks, maybe five gentle pats followed by one a little bit harder, then a pause, then the same again. When she starts to get warm I step it up to a faster rhythm, maybe with two harder smacks, and so on, until she's getting a full-on spanking that would make her run a mile if I'd started that way. That can take ten, even twenty minutes."

"So patience is obviously very important, and putting her pleasure before your own?"

"Yes. Not that I mind having a girl's bottom to play with."

"Well, no. May I have some examples please? How about the first time you spanked a girl, especially if it was also her first?"

"Yes, it was. That was fifteen years ago now, although I'd dreamt about spanking all my life. She was a musician, like me. We were doing a concert together out of town and I drove her back. We'd been flirting all the time, and on the way back I was teasing her by telling her she deserved a spanking for being such a flirt, and telling her that she ought to be spanked anyway, just for having such a lovely bottom. She dared me to do it, and so I did. We turned into a lane and I parked out of sight of the main road, where I thought it would be private enough. She was next to me in the front seat, so I pulled her across my lap. It was all a bit awkward, and it took me a while to get her trousers and knickers down, but she was very helpful. I spanked her bare, like that, with her bottom lifted so that anybody who came past would have seen her bare and that she was getting a spanking. She loved that, and I spent ages on her bottom and played with her until she came. That showed me how spanking makes delicious foreplay for both parties."

215

"So when you spank a girl you like to make her come?"

"Oh yes. Spanking brings girls, and men, into a lifted state. It makes you feel more sexual and I love to see a girl react that way."

"You seem very giving as a spanker, and not really concerned with dominance or punishment, even in a playful way?"

"Yes. It's not so much a dominant thing for me as a sensual one. My pleasure comes from the girl's excitement. I am assertive though, when I'm the one doing the spanking, and I like people to be assertive with me when I'm the one being spanked."

"Okay, so among the thirty-three girls you've given their first spankings, do you have a favourite, or perhaps an experience you'd particularly like to share?"

"Yes. Ellie. She was a nurse. I met her in a club and we became friends, but while she loved to watch me spank other people, she would never try it herself. Every time we were at a party together I'd try to persuade her but she'd always refuse, until it had become a bit of joke between us. It must have been more than a year before I turned up at a club to find her dressed as an adult schoolgirl, you know the style, a white blouse with a tie half undone, a pleated navy blue skirt with big white knickers underneath, little black shoes and over-the-knee socks. They don't call them over-the-knee socks for nothing!"

"I take it that's where she ended up?"

"No, I did her over a spanking bench, after spending most of the evening persuading her that dressing up as a naughty schoolgirl meant she definitely needed spanking, and probably wanted it deep down. Eventually she agreed, but made me promise to be very gentle with her. I was, but the good thing was that as we already knew each other so well it was up with her skirt and down with her knickers straight away, so I had a lovely bare little target right from the start. Picture her kneeling over the spanking stool like that, with her school skirt turned up and her big white knickers pulled down."

"I am, believe me. What was her figure like?"

"Quite tall, very slim, with long legs and a little round bottom."

"You seem to like very slim girls; Sophie, Kirsten, in fact nearly all those I've met."

"I'm not fussy, really, but I do love the way slim girls can't hide anything. When a slim girl bends over she shows everything, even if she keeps her legs together. Ellie was certainly showing everything and I could see she was wet even before I'd started. I was still very gentle, using my favourite rhythm of five little pats and then a sharp smack to very slowly warm her bottom. She was very quiet at first, not even answering me back when I bent down to talk to her, so I took it even more slowly than usual to let her get her head around what I was doing to her. Her body wanted it though and her body won out in the end. I have never seen a girl so wet from spanking, and when her bottom was a delicious cherry red all over I bent down and whispered into her ear again, asking if a naughty schoolgirl like her deserved the cane. She said she did, so I gave her two strokes, and then when she stayed down, two more, and another two. I usually stick to six-of-the-best but she obviously didn't want to get up, so I took it right up to a dozen, and that was when she asked for two across the backs of her thighs, which really hurts. I don't normally cane girls' thighs, but as she'd asked for it she got it, two hard strokes that left bright red lines in her flesh, just below where her bottom and thighs meet. With the second stroke she gave a sudden jerk and a little gasp, not from the pain, but because she'd come."

The Stats

I DON'T CLAIM THAT this book is an in-depth survey of first-time spankings, or even that it's representative. Most spankings are domestic, strictly play between partners and never revealed to the outside world, while in any event the fifty accounts I've recorded aren't nearly enough to yield statistically significant figures. Nevertheless, the book does give a genuine cross-section of erotic spankings and some things do stand out, both because they illuminate the world of spanking play and because go against popular myths about spanking.

Myth No 1 – Spanking is all about dirty old men abusing vulnerable women.

Every single spanking included in this book was consensual, so that doesn't tell us anything, but what is interesting is that of the fifty girls whose accounts I've recorded, thirty-five (70%), had a strong desire for erotic spanking before they received it. I didn't record how many of the women had enjoyed spankings from other women, but it's certainly the great majority, while nine (18%) had taken their first spanking from another women.

Myth No 2 – Women only accept spankings for money.

This is patently untrue. Any girl who is into spanking is sure to get offers of money for her services, and yet of the fifty girls in this book only fifteen (30%) have ever accepted money to be spanked. Of those fifteen, eleven (73%) had a strong desire for spanking before they received it. Only three (6%) of the women support themselves as sex workers, while most are now either professionals or housewives, with comparatively few in clerical or manual work.

Myth No 3 – Spanking is only for the decadent and the depraved.

If this was the case you'd expect the majority of my accounts to be from older women who've had a lot of sexual experience. In practice, twenty-eight (56%) had been spanked by the time they were twenty years old, and of those twenty-eight, seventeen (61%) were the instigators of their own first spanking.